PRAISE FOR *GERMS ARE NOT OUR ENEMY*

"In *Germs Are Not Our Enemy*, Marizelle Arce pinpoints the true causes of diseases—toxins, injury, and malnutrition. Germs are the innocent bystanders, often playing a useful role by cleaning up diseased tissue. Dr. Arce's work is an important contribution to our understanding of what makes us sick and how to stay well."
SALLY FALLON MORELL, President,
The Weston A. Price Foundation

"This book is very important as an updated and modern view into the terrain paradigm and pleomorphism which was needed."
JOSH BIGELSEN, cofounder of Bigelsen Academy

"Dr. Marizelle Arce has synthesized her many years of research and study with her practical experience to provide a comprehensive view of the terrain model that is highly readable. She interweaves history with modern findings to bring the reader to a clear understanding of why, as her title proclaims, 'germs' are not our enemy.

"Introducing readers to the work of many pioneers in their fields who have contributed to this body of knowledge, Marizelle helps us gain a recognition of the fundamental living entities that are ubiquitous. She refers to these entities appropriately as 'precursors' and explains how they trans-form themselves into the various forms we are repeatedly told are 'dangerous germs,' but which are, in fact, essential components that play important roles in the health of our bodies."

DAWN LESTER, coauthor of *What Really Makes You Ill?*

"As someone who has spent decades immersed in the terrain model of health, I found *Germs Are Not Our Enemy* to be a refreshing and powerful contribution to the conversation. Marizelle Arce doesn't just challenge the germ theory—she brings it all into context. I really appreciate her incorporating the historical roots of terrain medicine alongside her real-world, hands-on experience with patients. That kind of grounded wisdom is not common these days. Her connection to regenerative farming and permaculture reinforces the truth that health is inseparable from the land beneath our feet and the balance within our bodies."

ADAM BIGELSEN, terrain health educator, cofounder of Bigelsen Academy and the University of Terrain

GERMS ARE NOT OUR ENEMY

WHY THE NEW TERRAIN MEDICINE IS BEST FOR OPTIMAL HEALTH

MARIZELLE ARCE, N.D.

FOREWORD BY CHRISTIANE NORTHRUP, M.D.

ARCEBEL PRESS
Mount Vernon, New York

www.germsarenotourenemy.com

Cover design by Louis Belchou
Editing and book production by Stephanie Gunning

Germs Are Not Our Enemy / Marizelle Arce — 1st edition

Library of Congress Number 2025908316

ISBN 979-8-9926285-0-0 (paperback)
ISBN 979-8-9926285-2-4 (epub)

DISCLAIMER

This book contains the opinions and general thoughts of the author. The information and advice in the book is intended only as general guidelines for reference. The book is by no means intended as a substitute for the medical advice of the reader's personal physician. The reader should regularly consult a physician in matters relating to his/her health or as pertains to any advice related to exercise, diet, supplements, homeopathy, sleep, personal health, or any other assistance. Specifically, a qualified physician should be consulted with respect to any symptoms that may require diagnosis or medical attention. The authors, editors, and publishers accept no liability for any injury arising out of the use of the material contained herein, and make no warranty, express or implied, with respect to the contents of this publication.

TO MY DAUGHTERS AND THE FUTURE OF HUMANITY.

VITAM IMPENDERE VERO.

CONTENTS

FOREWORD BY
CHRISTIANE NORTHRUP, M.D. *page xiii*

PREFACE *page xix*

INTRODUCTION *page xxiii*

PART I. THE HISTORY YOU DIDN'T KNOW

CHAPTER 1. *page 3*
The Discovery of "Germs"

CHAPTER 2. *page 21*
The Main Contention of Germ Theory

CHAPTER 3. *page 35*
The Neglected Terrain Model of
Health and Healing

CHAPTER 4. *page 61*
Early Views of Microbes

CHAPTER 5. *page 81*
The Key to Optimal Health

CHAPTER 6. *page 111*
The Importance of the Environment to Our Terrain

CHAPTER 7. *page 133*
How Do Viruses Fit the Terrain Model?

CHAPTER 8. *page 147*
The Flaw of Modern Medicine and Its Industrialization

PART II. THE BETTER WAY TO CREATE OPTIMAL HEALTH

CHAPTER 9. *page 167*
Keeping the Balance of the Terrain

CHAPTER 10. *page 181*
Terrain-Model Therapeutics

CHAPTER 11. *page 195*
Overcoming Malnutrition Caused by Deficits in Our Farming Practices

CHAPTER 12. *page 217*
Detoxification and Reducing the Body's Workload

CHAPTER 13 *page 233*
You Are the Inheritor of Your Ancestors' Microbiomes and Terrain

CHAPTER 14 *page 253*
Break the Spell of Germ Theory Everywhere

AFTERWORD *page 273*
Evolve Your Health and Your Health-Care Options

ACKNOWLEDGMENTS *page 283*

NOTES *page 287*

RESOURCES *page 305*

ABOUT THE AUTHOR *page 306*

FOREWORD

I want you to take a moment and ask yourself the following question: How much easier would my life be if I never again worried about germs or "catching" something from someone else—on a plane, in a class, in a movie theater, or a family gathering? What if you knew you could trust your terrain and your immune system to do what it was designed to do, keep you healthy, because you know how to keep your terrain healthy?

Well, that is exactly what you are going to learn how to do in this brilliantly researched book that debunks pretty much everything you've ever been taught about germs and your health—and replaces those beliefs with empowering knowledge that you can apply right now to keep yourself healthy for a lifetime.

Of course, this flies in the face of everyday life. Here's an example. One of my colleagues called me today to say that he wouldn't be able to come to an event we were planning in which we were showing the movie *The Biggest Little Farm*—about soil health, organic agriculture, and the balance of nature. A classic example of healthy terrain in action. He said he had the flu and didn't want to "give" it to anyone else.

I wasn't going to argue with him about the fact that you actually cannot "give" anyone the flu. After all, most of us have had decades of indoctrination—beginning in childhood—

about avoiding people with colds or flu lest we "catch" that same cold.

Well, guess what? Hundreds of studies have documented the fact that you actually cannot "catch" a cold.

Interestingly, during the great Spanish flu epidemic of 1918, they tried to infect healthy people with the excretions of those who were sick. And no matter what they sprayed in their throats or injected them with, they couldn't make them sick.

So what actually caused so many people to get sick back then? First of all, the death toll was far lower than we have been told. My colleague Lee Merritt, M.D., went back to the old newspapers and discovered that fact. First-person accounts from that time reported that those who wore masks and were injected with vaccines of the period were the first to get sick.

But there was something else going on: a change in the electromagnetic field around people. We are, after all, energetic creatures who are sensitive to electromagnetic frequencies, such as sun spots and radiation from cell towers and microwave radiation. There is ample evidence that the real cause of the Spanish flu deaths was the electrification of the earth via the telegraph lines.

My colleague Thomas S. Cowan, M.D., who wrote *The Contagion Myth*, had this to say in an interview during the COVID pandemic:

> *In 1918 after the biggest pandemic, the Spanish flu pandemic of 1918,* [Rudolf] *Steiner was asked what was*

> *all this about. And he said, "Well, viruses are simply excretions of a toxic cell. Viruses are pieces of DNA or RNA with a few other proteins they brought out from the cell. They happen when the cell is poisoned. They are not the cause of anything."*
>
> *Every pandemic in the last 150 years there was a quantum leap in the electrification of the earth. In 1918, late fall of 1917, there was the introduction of radio waves around the world. Whenever you expose any biological system to a new electromagnetic field you poison it, you kill some and the rest go into a kind of suspended animation so that interestingly they live a little bit longer and sicker.*[1]

I have a friend in his eighties whose grandfather's job was to travel around Maine on behalf of the railroad. This man documented the fact that many of the telegraph operators of those days died of sudden cardiac arrests.

Despite evidence to the contrary, most people have been thoroughly indoctrinated into the belief that it is germs—not environmental terrain factors—that cause sickness. Most stubbornly hold on to this belief with religious fervor, thus denying themselves and their immune systems the benefits of the liberating knowledge so brilliantly outlined in this book. No matter how much information you provide to the contrary, many will argue that they got sick because "everyone at the party was sick" or " I was at a superspreader event." It is little wonder that it was so easy to convince so many people all over the planet to get a dangerous, fast-tracked experimental biologic injected into them during the COVID years from 2020 to 2025. This would never have happened had they been well educated about how to keep their terrain healthy.

As a holistic obstetrician/gynecologist and author of three *New York Times* bestselling books on women's health, I have long known about the debate between Louis Pasteur ("It's the germ that causes the disease") and his contemporary Antoine Béchamp ("It's the terrain in which the germ finds itself that determines the whether or not a person gets sick"). As it turns out—and is so aptly proven in the pages of this brilliant book—Béchamp was correct. But Pasteur was a better marketer. And his approach to eradicating "germs" with drugs and vaccines was far more profitable than upgrading the terrain—which requires lifestyle changes.

This kind of history has repeated itself over and over again—generally at the expense of the general public vs those who are making a profit. Let's take Thomas Edison vs. Nicola Tesla. Tesla's work demonstrated that alternating current not only worked better, but it also could have provided free energy for humanity. Edison, on the other hand, promoted direct current and was backed by individuals intent on making money.

No wonder they called one of the major electric companies of the day Con Edison! Meanwhile, Tesla's lab was ransacked and his inventions kept from the public.

We are now at a crossroads in our understanding of health and disease. We've gone as far as we can go with the current approach. We must heed the words of Jeff Goldblum's character Dr. Ian Malcolm in the famous movie *Jurassic Park.* Upon hearing the footsteps of a giant prehistoric creature on the island that was home to Jurassic Park, Malcolm is told, "Don't worry. They are all females."

Malcolm replies, "Nature always finds a way."

And indeed this is true. The more we tinker with the balance of nature, the more problems we create. The harder we fight germs with powerful drugs, the stronger those germs become. Hence, we now have antibiotic resistant superbugs in many hospitals that ever more powerful antibiotics cannot touch. And despite the fact that the CDC-recommended vaccine schedule is now up to seventy-two shots by the age of eighteen, 54 percent of our children now have a chronic disease.

The only answer to our current health crises is to shore up our terrain. And quickly. We become resilient and healthy humans only when we embrace the fact that our bodies are comprised of vast communities of microbes that are designed to live together in balance and harmony unless something in our diets, beliefs, or lifestyles tips us out of balance. And that is precisely what you will learn how to do in *Germs are Not Our Enemy.*

So, dive in and learn what it takes to be healthy. The only thing you have to lose is your fear of germs!

Christiane Northrup, M.D.,
Bestselling author of *Women's Bodies, Women's Wisdom, The Wisdom of Menopause,* and *Goddesses Never Age*

PREFACE

When I was in naturopathic medical school, I saw a post about a job opening for some sort of sales rep for a company based in Europe that sold homeopathic and isopathic products. Needing to make money and wanting to learn to do something health-related outside of school, this notice caught my eye. I did a bit of research on the company and became very interested. The company, Pleo Sanum, manufactured products designed by Gunther Enderlein, Ph.D., a German zoologist who believed that the organisms living in the human body change shape based on changes in the environment of the body, a phenomenon known as *pleomorphism.* Studying them through a microscope, Dr. Enderlein was able to discern that bacteria and fungi will alter their appearance under certain toxic conditions. He also observed these same micro-organisms forming from what he deemed to be their precursors in the body, which he named *protits.* The protits would assume the form of a bacterium or a fungus based on what was happening in the environment in which the microorganism resided, such as in the blood or the gut.

As I dug deeper into Enderlein's research and ideas about wellness before my interview, I started believing that the germ theory which is the underpinning of much of the conventional medical treatment we in the United States receive—especially the idea of "one germ, one disease" —is a fabrication.

From what I could tell as an outsider, the staff of Pleo Sanum were boldly proposing that the manifestation of all diseases, aside from those resulting from trauma or exposure to toxic substances, is based on the condition of the environment *inside* the body. That diseases aren't "caught" from microbes outside the body. That microbes like bacteria and fungi are products of the changing of the environment *within the body.* And that they *pleomorph*, or alter themselves, into forms appropriate for survival in a new environment.

When I went for an interview for the sales job at Pleo Sanum, I am certain that I was not what the interviewer expected. My attire was relaxed and sloppy. I wasn't freshly showered, so I must have looked like I'd just fallen out of bed. But I walked into the interview room carrying a stack of research folders containing articles by Enderlein and members of his company that I'd highlighted. Within the first fifteen minutes, I was hired, though I wasn't told this until after the ninety-minute interview was over. My obsession with Enderlein's work and all the "new" science I'd learned, absorbed, and reiterated captivated my interviewer, and he saw that I was thoroughly passionate about my new endeavor. He wound up being my mentor later on.

My position as a rep for Pleo Sanum afforded me the opportunity to teach other students of naturopathy about the fundamentals of health destruction, as well as how to utilize the homeopathic and isopathic remedies the company made. Being that I was accomplished in teaching students, my title was changed to Medical Support Associate, and I was encouraged to reach further afield and teach doctors, nurses, chiropractors, and other professionals outside of my school about the products. The more I learned, trained, and taught about Pleo Sanum's ideology, the more I understood about the terrain of the human body and how farfetched the theory of germs is which underpins much of conventional medical practice.

My education in terrain medicine didn't stop there. During my first year as a sales rep, I attended several conventions and seminars where I was able to engage with other naturopathic practitioners like me as well as with biologists and other types of scientists who agree that the germ theory of conventional medicine is false, largely based upon their own studies, practices, and experience of workings with individual patients for decades. Each of these professionals understood that natural medicine is really about supporting the body's well-being and homeostatic mechanisms rather than about "attacking" germs.

At one of those early conventions, I happened upon the book *Politics in Healing* by Daniel Haley. In it, every chapter is devoted to describing a different solution or treatment that someone came up with which mainstream medicine viewed as quackery or fraudulent even though it had helped thousands of people rid themselves of an infection or a disease—even cancer. In one chapter, he writes about other scientists who proved, just as Enderlein did, that not only will bacteria and fungi transform themselves into different shapes and types of organism, but they also come from super tiny precursors within the body. Though I had already been exposed to this information, seeing it reiterated by Haley made my world seem frighteningly small.

How did I get through my life until then not knowing that not only was there one scientist who thought the one germ-one disease theory of contagions was a load of garbage, but there were several—maybe even hundreds—of scientists, doctors, and wellness advocates who believed the same?

After experiencing the implosion of information I had formerly relied upon, I realized that my job and my life goal were to connect what I had recently learned to everything I had been taught during my schooling. That was when the implosion turned into a learning explosion.

No more was there a fear of "catching" or "infecting." It was time for me to focus on means for keeping the body healthy. That led me to become aware of the grand importance of nutrition and building the body's resources to vast heights. I studied the works of many great individuals, like the dentists and nutrition pioneers Weston A. Price, D.D.S., and Royal Lee, D.D.S., and the father of North American naturopathy Benedict Lust, N.D., made sense.

Everything was clear ultimately. Food is the real medicine. Toxins and trauma that alter our bodies' terrain are the real sources of disease.

INTRODUCTION

"You have been educated to believe disease is an entity—that it is a specific something that you can 'catch' or contract by exposure to some virulent germ or some person or thing that is harboring such germs. Before I finish, I shall prove the fallacy of this theory and the fallacy of such an education."
STANFORD CLAUNCH, N.D.

Naturopathic doctors are committed to using the least invasive, least toxic methods to help our patients. Holistically oriented, we base our work on the concept of *terrain* and believe in the inherent power of the body to heal itself. This means we look at everything going on in and around the individuals we're treating, viewing the internal and external environment of a person as a landscape of exchange that must be healthy in its entirety for these people to stay well. Our focus is on developing optimal health and symbiosis within our bodies by integrating natural therapies with modern tools. *Germs Are Not Our Enemy* will introduce you to this approach. I anticipate this book reaching a professional audience, a self-care audience, and a parenting audience, among others.

Microbes live in us and around us, on our skin, in our guts, and in the air, water, and soil of our natural environment, yet we've been taught by medicine to fear them. We've been told that they make us sick, that their presence is the cause of diseases rather than an outcome of what is seen as disease. Really it's a sign that a rebalancing process has already occurred while the body was reestablishing its health and restoring its homeostasis. In *Germs Are Not Our Enemy: Why the New Terrain Medicine Is Best for Optimal Health*, I will explain why "germs" are not what people commonly believe them to be. Not our enemy. Then I will posit an alternative, supportive approach to health and healing that is a better way than conventional medicine, which relies overmuch on toxic chemicals and invasive practices.

Bottom-line, Louis Pasteur got it wrong.

Naturopathic medicine is an old-fashioned (in the best sense of the term), common-sense approach to strengthening the body's innate resources and homeostatic balancing mechanisms so poor health does not occur. The core idea is that if we support the body in meeting its needs, the body can overcome its challenges. Until the twentieth-century, naturopathic practitioners were recognized as the peers of medical doctors and osteopaths in the United States and worked in the same institutions. But American culture, being dominated by corporate interests, has a fondness for overriding nature with technology and synthetic substances that can be patented and sold. Our medical and pharmaceutical system became such a big business that physicians treating people by promoting a healthy lifestyle based on good nutrition, clean water and air, sleep, and other routines that are just being remembered now—because we desperately need them—were pushed to the side.

Today, more and more people in the United States and other industrially developed nations are clamoring for a change that brings us back into harmony with nature. This book will reveal a path to freedom through harmony, which begins by restoring suppressed knowledge about what makes us sick and how we stay well. Health experts, parents, and wellness enthusiasts all want the madness to stop.

There are a lot of people feeling afraid for their lives because of public policies that were enacted during 2020 and 2021 and messages that indicated they should feel threatened. There are also a lot of people feeling fed up and angry because they believe they've been lied to by an overly controlling government and subjected against their will to efforts by a medical system that is pushing bad and dangerous products on them in pursuit of profits. If you are one of these people, I wrote *Germs Are Not the Enemy* for you.

Nature is around and within us. To honor and support our inherent healing mechanisms, we must first shift the mindset and attitudes that get in the way of doing what is best for our bodies. Why do some people become symptomatic when supposedly exposed to microbes and others do not? Because good health boils down to having an internal terrain that is balanced and regenerative. Poor health results from imbalanced terrain. A balanced terrain is the most important factor in how well we feel.

The new terrain medicine takes advantage of contemporary tools that can help us analyze the functionality and symbiosis of the body, including the blood, looking for physical and emotional imbalances and the presence of toxins. But in many ways, its essential practices are quite similar to those of the medicine of our forebearers in the late nineteenth and early twentieth centuries. Science has advanced in its ability to peer into the microscopic world. So, it is now time to correct the mistakes we've made in our society based on wrong information.

Terrain medicine is built on recognition that human health and the health of the world are integrally linked in every regard. Our bodies are one with the environment that surrounds them.

"I believe that Nature Cure people are right when they apply to physical disease the same method that we apply to psychical disease. Just as a buried wish should be lived out, so should a buried poison be allowed to find its way out."

JAMES C. THOMSON, SR.

"Human beings, the potentially highest form of life expression on this planet, have built the vast pharmaceutical industry for the central purpose of poisoning the lowest form of life on the planet—germs! One of the biggest tragedies of human civilization is the precedence of chemicals over nutrition."

RICHARD MURRAY, N.D.

PART I

THE HISTORY YOU DIDN'T KNOW

ONE

□□□□□□□□

THE DISCOVERY OF "GERMS"

"Most secrets of knowledge have been discovered by plain and neglected men than by men of popular fame. And this is so with good reason. For the men of popular fame are busy on popular matters."
ROGER BACON

Since the late nineteenth century, all medicine and almost all biological science has been dominated by the premise that disease is related to our exposure to germs. Therefore it is common to believe that we "contract" or "catch" diseases. Treated as a law, this theory has altered how doctors and scientists view, treat, and remove disease elements. Until very recently, the notion that the body is innately sterile and can be made to harbor only "good" and beneficial microorganisms has been pushed as a universal solution for health questions. But historically, most physicians, and science in general, understood that if some-one became ill, then something had disrupted their body's systems and was interfering with its internal homeostatic environment.

Physiologically speaking, *homeostasis* is a "self-regulating process by which biological systems maintain stability while adjusting to changing external conditions."[1] Harvard professor of physiology Walter Cannon (1871–1945) coined the phrase to describe the tendency of the body to return to equilibrium following stress. For example, our hearts beat faster when we run. But after stopping, the heartrate slows of its own accord. This is homeostasis in operation.

The corruption of the historic doctrine of disruption with the false hypothesis of invading, contagious *bugs*—a term used to refer to all kinds of microorganisms found in and on our bodies and in the air, water, and soil of our planet—almost entirely destroyed humanity's common understanding of the synergistic connection we have both with each other and with the nature that resides in and outside of us.

The actual failure of germ theory to prevent or cure the diseases that ail us has not only created concern and unending questions in the minds of laypeople, but has allowed for the formation of innumerable money-making industries that flourish from the battle between human and microbe. No other theory has pervasively embedded itself in almost everything we do at the level of the human experience. And because of the disconnect science has created with how it views the body, we continue to create more questions that the germ theory cannot answer.

Everyone knows the name Louis Pasteur. His surname is embedded in the word *pasteurized* that is printed on the labels of milk cartons and cheese. It is forever linked to a fundamental system of thinking that every scientist is taught: the germ theory. Although Pasteur did not himself discover bacteria or viruses, his love of science combined with his ambitious nature put a deep, irreversible dent into the biology we are taught today. Robert Koch, another pioneer of the germ theory during Pasteur's era, created a tarnished gold standard that members of the fields of microbiology and medicine still follow to this day, although his methodologies are being questioned by our contemporaries. Before Pasteur and Koch, various men of antiquity had built the shaky foundation that they stood on, only reinforcing how frail their theory really is.

Modern medicine took the Pasteurian hypothesis that germs make people sick and built a house of cards with it that has started to crumble under the weight of more and more sick people not being helped. To understand why the practice of medicine has gone so far astray, we need to take a step back into the past and witness the events that have led us to our current situation.

My Awakening

As a child, I wanted to become a doctor despite the fact that doctors and their medications rarely provided me with answers or cures. I was frequently put on an antibiotic or given an antihistamine or something intended to halt a constant infection in my throat, ears, nose, or stomach. Regardless, I still wanted to be a doctor, but not the kind I was used to seeing. From the very beginning, I could see that medicine had inconsistencies.

I never once thought of entering the field of medicine in order to treat my own condition. I went into medicine because I was enamored. I was in love with the idea of helping people and truly giving them the answers and solutions they were seeking. But the moment I began my studies at an allopathic medical school—an institution that teaches conventional medicine—the inconsistencies I'd pushed aside earlier came roaring back in my face.

I distinctly remembered how I always wound up with a vaginal yeast infection when taking an antibiotic for a sinus infection, and how almost everyone else I knew did as well. I also discovered that I wasn't the only student in school questioning modern medicine. I had friends, even professors, who had some sort of health or medical issue whose symptoms modern medicine was merely suppressing, rather than healing. This failure to cure led me to dive deeper into anthropology, seeking missing insights. What might traditional healers have known?

In the course of my research, I was fortunate to come upon the works of Drs. Weston A. Price and Royal Lee, dentists who became advocates of healthy nutrition. In the early twentieth century, dentists were like nutritionists and helped people connect the dots between diet and lifestyle and the way the body will display neglect through the teeth.

But these two particular doctors of dentistry took their research to the next level, by identifying how industrialism, with its poisons and processed foods, and the disconnected medical establishment, prescribing their quick fixes of chemical-based medicines, were the root causes of many, if not all, the ails of society. They traveled the world and saw firsthand how the people of many traditional cultures with nutritionally rich diets, natural living, and little to no medical care, had robust bodies, beautiful dentition, and no diseases of which to speak.

I had a blossoming of ideas derived from the research of Price and Lee, including the realization that modern medicine lacks a significant piece of the health puzzle. The holistic health industry tries to fill in the gaps of knowledge, though it falls short.

Miasma Theory

From my reading, I discerned that for much of the nineteenth century, along with almost all of written history prior, sickness was thought to be caused by bad air, water, or soil. This theory of disease is the *miasmatic theory* or the *miasma theory*. To be accurate, some people also believed that a demon was affecting the body or magic was involved in the creation of various conditions—epilepsy or Tourette's syndrome, for example—a nonsensical idea to be sure.

The miasma theory holds that disease comes from exposure to "bad air" emanating from something rotten or putrid, such as decomposing foods, which people believed were releasing poisonous fumes.

Many cultures have had notions about the environment's role in influencing a person's health. Illness was rarely seen as communicable. Instead, it was believed that exposure to poison was linked to there being a multitude of "infected" people. From antiquity to the Middle Ages, a number of writers attributed the spread of many diseases to the mists of toxic air from either marshes or mountain tops. An 1854 cholera epidemic in London, for instance, was believed to originate from putrid water of the Thames River, although a man named John Snow tried to prove otherwise.[2]

Waterborne contamination was commonplace because there was no indoor plumbing yet, also being that hygiene and sanitation were not practiced for centuries in congested towns and kingdoms. The people of ancient China and other Asian cultures produced well-documented accounts of diseases manifesting from contaminated air. Yet, once in a while, a researcher would come along to explain that perhaps something unseen in the air was actually causing the problem.

The "Seed" or Germ

In the early sixteenth century, Girolamo Fracastoro wrote a treatise on how invisible seeds in the wind, which he named *seminaria*, were the cause of illness. In the seventeenth century, when plague was running rampant, Jesuit scholar Athanasius Kircher, Pierre Borel (physician to King Louis

XIV of France), and Italian parasitologist Francesco Redi (who had done observations of maggots in putrid meat) furthered that belief with their findings of "little animals" living in the air or within other animals. This was during the same period in the late 1600s as when Antoni Van Leeuwenhoek, a self-taught scientist and one of the inventors of the microscope, discovered *little animals*, as he too called them, within the tartar of his teeth, under the lens of his self-constructed machine. But his observations told nothing of their behavior.[3]

Once the microscope was developed, it allowed researchers to peer inside the world of tiny microbes and make assumptions about what they saw concerning disease; this furthered theories of contagion. This was the start of the "a germ is a seed of a disease" idea first recorded in 1796.

Slovenian physician Marcus A. Plenciz presented the earliest theory that resembles the current contagion-germ model. Later, German pathologist Frederich Henle further developed the thesis of microorganisms causing disease, which Robert Koch, a famous student of his, who won the Nobel Prize in 1905 for his work on tuberculosis, would eventually expand upon.[4] Koch is considered one of the founders of the field of bacteriology.

Edward Jenner and the First "Vaccine"

English doctor Edward Jenner, in the late 1700s, developed an idea for prevention of smallpox based on the mere superstition that milkmaids who had blisters on their hands (aka cowpox) never developed smallpox. Since Leeuwenhoek's time, inoculation, which they called *ingrafting* at the time, was done supposedly to deter the severe effects of a disease.[5]

More than anything, this technique specifically was seen to be the *cause of* the epidemics since it was the application of someone's sickly blood being pushed into a deep wound of another person, and that it was also well-known. Jenner used this same technique of ingrafting, and instead of using blood from a smallpox patient, he utilized the liquid from milkmaids blisters to "vaccinate" a boy. It supposedly worked—the technique spread far and wide, and by 1802, it was believed and sensationalized that smallpox was limited in its outbreaks.

The word *vaccine* derives from the Latin word for cow, *vacca.*

On further examination of the competing treatment of smallpox during that time, the treatments utilized in the cities and newly colonized towns consisted of an oatmeal gruel, cooked fruits, liquor, emetic wines, and blood-letting, while doctors in country villages prescribed soups, boiled milk, and bed rest.[6] No wonder milkmaids in the country didn't ever get smallpox!

The natural down trend of smallpox along with better hygiene in a multitude of locations all over the world contributed to the reduced smallpox outbreaks. Yet no one confirmed this under a microscope and few trusted the new vaccine. It took until the middle of the nineteenth century for the microscope revival and microorganism research to begin again.

Louis Pasteur and Robert Koch

Considered the foremost modern proponent of germ theory, chemist Louis Pasteur first studied crystals using the microscope. This research led him to study fermentation. The work of French physicist Joseph Gay-Lussac caught his eye. Gay-Lussac filled a test tube with sterilized crushed grapes and covered it with liquid mercury. No fermentation occurred, which was contrary to the expedience with which fermentation occurred in wine barrels. The moment oxygen was introduced to the grape mush under the mercury, however, fermentation started. Although Gay-Lussac could not reproduce the experiment consistently, he contended that the key factor was the oxygen.[7]

Other scientists, including Pasteur, disagreed. They erroneously believed that an organism in the air causes fermentation. In fact, fermentation is a metabolic process that occurs in a few different ways, most of them occurring outside of the presence of oxygen. Although it was believed, at that time, that it was the air contaminating the sample, the microorganisms present in a fermented material are there because of *spontaneous generation*. Essentially these organisms arise from *within* the substance as it is fermented. Fermentation is a decomposition process, which is aided by the microbes.

Despite Pasteur not being able to adequately disprove the evidence of spontaneous generation, he continued to assert that tissues whether human, animal or plant, were sterile and that microbes in the air would come into contaminating it.[8] He founded and based his idea of airborne germs on an experiment he did that was published in the *Annales de Chimie et de Physique*, that stated that he was able to create a ferment, like yeast in a medium with just air exposure and not with any living substance! All scientists to date know that this is impossible, making that experiment a fake one.

As we know, this unfounded belief led Pasteur to develop *pasteurization*, a method to prevent the spoilage of wine and beer. All his experiments demonstrated that bacteria were found in fermentation and putrefaction. However, he was *never* able to produce these same creatures—bacteria—in experiments on *living tissue*. In a public lecture in 1911 in London, "Pasteur, the Plagiarist," Montague Richard Leverson, M.D., reported how in an experiment that Pasteur once referenced as *famous*, Pasteur had claimed "to have proved that fragments which had been parts of living bodies were safe from change or putrefaction . . . . and yet in his own description of that experiment, while asserting that no air-borne germs had reached it, and that no putrefactive or other change had taken place, he described it as becoming *gamey*, and was too ignorant to perceive that this effect, itself a step on the road to putrefaction."[9]

In another experiment of blood, Pasteur described changes in the blood, such as coagulation and crystallization, yet concluded the blood was sterile. So, clearly he was misinterpreting his data. His misguided conclusion that germs cause contagions led him to continue finding ways to remove the bacteria from beverages instead of addressing and understanding the materials in which they were found—their *terrain*.

In other words, bacteria weren't *causing* the degradation in the wine and beer; they were present in the wine and beer *because* the wine and beer were decomposing.

Translating this idea to the human body, my view as a terrain doctor is that when we see bacteria in living tissue, like we would in a cut on a leg that appears red and swollen, the bacteria are not causing the inflammation around the wound; rather, they are there to support the body in responding to the injury and devastation to the various tissues.

Pasteur's own work could not provide evidence for his theory of pathological transmission of disease, of contagion! "Pasteur believed that if milk, grapes, and butter fermented due to living organisms . . . ," these same creations would create diseases of the body.[10] It is here that Pasteur has actually proved the terrain paradigm: when milk ages, it produces lactic acid by way of endogenous bacteria. When crushed grapes get old, same thing, and the product is alcohol. Same with aged butter growing mold. So if we analyze this pattern, follow this premise of thinking, we see that when something has degenerated and is decomposing, intrinsically it is broken down, just as we are from our own microbiome, making space for new tissue to regenerate in that space.

Regardless, Pasteur published his observations as the *vegetable or fungus germ theory of disease.* Support began to accrue for this theory in the late nineteenth century, and by 1870, Louis Pasteur was already well on his way to being a national hero in France, especially for his creation of a rabies vaccine. The irony of this is that, at that time, "rabies [was] a rare disease that killed fewer than one hundred people in France every year. Most people bitten by rabid animals do not develop the disease; most of those 'saved' by Pasteur were not even doomed from the outset."[11]

Additionally, within Pasteur's notes he admits that his research led him to "inconclusive and frustrating results."[12] He did establish that "research on rabies had been impeded by the fact that the disease was not consistently transmitted either by the injection of rabid saliva or the bite of a rabid animal. More surprisingly, since it seemed clear that the nervous system and especially the brain was the ultimate seat of the disease, even subcutaneous injections of rabid nervous tissue did not always transmit the disease from one animal to another."[13]

Biographers have tended to burnish Pasteur's reputation using less truth and more fabrication. His inconsistent findings laid the foundation for the approach to healing we now call *modern medicine.* It was Pasteur's self-promotion and constant assuagement of critics that helped him develop fame and promote his ideas. During his time, to speak against his theory was to be considered "unpatriotic" or "antiestablishment. But he didn't pull the wool over everyone's eyes. In unpublished manuscripts, Pasteur's colleague Claude Bernard criticized Pasteur and disapproved of his germ-causative theory of fermentation.

According to biographer Gerald L. Geison, most of Pasteur's findings were fraudulent and only enumerated in unpublished works he kept until his death. He stole experiments from both colleagues and adversaries.[14]

When a person compares Pasteur's work to one of his biggest rival, French chemist and physician Antoine Béchamp, M.D., Ph.D., you would find "full proof that the great god of the (supposedly) men of the latter half of the century, and of the many of the present, was in fact the most astonishing of plagiarists and distorters of other men's discoveries."[15]

Pasteur's journals have revealed how he was secretly injecting poisons into the brains and bodies of animals to ensure the outcome of many of his experiments went the way he hypothesized they would. Why did he keep secret his use of chemicals to attenuate microorganisms? Did he understand that these chemicals themselves were agents of the responses he saw in the body? Although he never tested the theory, Pasteur suggested that a disease might be controlled by exposing a wound to germ-killing chemicals. So what then was his obsession with inoculations?

While renowned medical institutions were supporting Pasteur's research, he discovered new facts that contradicted his previous observations. Through his efforts to create vaccinations and his attempts to diminish the virulency of microbes caused him to witness the variability of resistance to disease and the adaptive capacity of so-called germs. Through fermentation experiments alone, Pasteur came to realize that bacteria could be beneficial in certain contexts if controlled properly.

He also became aware that by attempting to change an organism's virulence, it, too, was able to adapt to different situations and environments, making Pasteur one of the first proponents for the phenomenon of *pleomorphism*, that was actually discovered concurrently by his lesser-known adversary Béchamp.[16]This discovery flew in the face of the germ theory of the day, which was in its infancy.

Physician and microbiologist Robert Koch, who was a German contemporary of Pasteur, took the reins from Pasteur and set out to develop a set of criteria—or postulates—for experimentation to explain disease and advance the discovery of microbes that he believed caused them. Like Pasteur, Koch believed that each specific organism created one specific disease and did not adapt, transform, or change in any way.[17]

Unlike Pasteur, he was a researcher who had specific, regimented ways of studying microorganisms. He had studied the procedures of many scientists of renown. This led to a rift between the two men, both wanting to be perceived as the founding father of the new science. Their distinct approaches to dealing with disease further fueled their rivalry. Pasteur believed in *controlling* the germs, while Koch emphasized *complete extermination.*

To curb the spread of diseases, Pasteur favored procedures like inoculations, even ones not fully evaluated.

Koch supported public education on hygiene and the use of serum therapy, scratching the skin of an inflicted person and rubbing a "serum" into the wound, as was done years before with milkmaids to prevent smallpox.

Due to Koch's work on the tuberculosis germ, his postulates became widely accepted by modern scientists. He hypothesized that a verifiably causative pathogen must be one that can be:

- Found in all cases of the disease being examined.
- Contained in a purified culture.
- Capable of producing the original infection when taken from the culture, even after several generations of the culture.
- Retrieved from any animal infected from the culture, and then cultured to show it is the same organism.

Many of Pasteur's experiments had failed to produce the same infection after several cultures. In fact, repeating cultures of microbes was how Pasteur created his rabies and anthrax vaccines—and he got diminished manifestations of these diseases after continuous culturing. Therefore, we know Pasteur could not follow Koch's postulates.

As time passed, Pasteur was not the only researcher whose experiments did not align with the postulates. Countless times, what was seen as pathogenicity (the ability of an organism to supposedly produce disease, and how intensely) substantially decreased when an organism was removed from the body and placed on a Petri dish.

As this type of experimentation continued, scientists made excuses for the lack of adherence to their revered postulates. Dogmatic scientists would try to justify the contradiction between their results and germ theory by insisting that a multitude of different bacteria can cause similar symptom patterns or types of infection. An example being the illness pneumonia, which has supposed fungal, bacterial, viral, alveolar, and interstitial forms.

But because of variations, there are a number of professionals in many fields of study today who disagree with Koch's postulates. They insist these rules are holding back advancement in the field of virology and other forms of study on the ultramicroscopic level. Specifically, leprosy and syphilis could never be grown in a pure culture medium, which added to the seed of doubt for the postulates.

Once exposed, the inconsistencies of germ theory inspired more scrutiny. Another scientist stepped in with his theory, Moldavian zoologist Ilya (Élie) Metchnikoff was jointly awarded the Noble Prize in Physiology in 1908 for identifying the process of phagocytosis in which white blood cells engulf foreign material that enters the body. His research laid the foundation for the new discipline of immunology.

Metchnikoff's work helped remove the doubt that many had about why some people become ill from exposure to germs, and some do not. But his findings did not sway the opinions of those who believed poor hygiene and sanitation—properties of external terrain—are more of the problem than the germs. Pathologist Rudolf Virchow, nurse and social reformer Florence Nightingale, and chemist Max von Pettenkofer, champions of improved social conditions, were not swayed by ideas of germ contagion.

TWO

□□□□□□□□□

THE MAIN CONTENTION OF GERM THEORY

"If the 'germ theory of disease' were correct, there'd be no one living to believe it."
BARTLETT JOSHUA PALMER, D.C.

The main contention of germ theory is that a single microbe causes each disease. The foundation of this one germ-one disease ideology is a blind faith in human beings as living above and apart from the rest of nature. A web of lies about invasion and contagion was woven over the past 120 years to reinforce a faulty view of the body as a machine that can be manipulated chemically. Anthropological observations from traditional societies experiencing less disease than the societies in developed countries and historical inaccuracies about diseases were swept under the rug if they were unsupportive of fearing contagion. Luckily, a few determined researchers stood up to proponents of the faulty science and proved that germ scientists missed a few things.

It is the contention of germ theory that sickness in our bodies is the result of healthy tissue being overrun by specific vicious, parasitic microbes that are breaking things down. These microbes either come from within us, and we're hosts to their supposed pathogenic ways due to variables in our immunity; or they are invaders from the outside, entering our bodies through various entrances and exits, like the mouth, the nose, or a cut on an arm. According to this theory, each microorganism has specific attributes of existence; therefore, certain ones can only be found in certain locations in the body—and under certain conditions.

Mainstream advocates of germ theory insist that each different microorganism creates a specific illness, producing a general set of symptoms that would affect most people on exposure, and that the microorganisms can be transmitted (depending on the type of organism it is) either through the air, contaminated materials, bodily fluids, or embryologically. This is the backbone belief behind contagiousness and the communicability of microorganisms.

Although only a theory, germ theory has long been touted as fact, and any person questioning it as such is seen as a deluded person of no importance. By this thinking, most diseases are caused by invasive microorganisms reproducing at rates that the body cannot manage. So, this type of thinking has led many people, if not most of the world, to fear microorganisms as invasive and pervasive regardless of their efforts at disinfection. School children are taught the bad deeds of these unfriendly organisms, while hospitals and healthcare facilities saturate their clinics with antiseptic substances.

Germophobia is augmented by institutions that are monetarily supporting research to find new or undiscovered "disease-producing" organisms.

I am personally skeptical of any research that is conducted without the regimented use of the scientific method. I am even more skeptical about research on microbes that is funded by institutions looking to profit off the sale of medications specifically created to kill microbes discovered by the research. Many germ scientists fail to use proper scientific methodology, although they pump out reports of newly discovered bacteria every year.

The *scientific method* is a well-recognized experimentation process through which reliable data are generated and empirically analyzed. Experiments must have controls and be designed to be reproducible in order to validate or disprove an initial hypothesis.

When the germ theory was being tested early on, many scientists formulated their hypotheses based on conclusions that they had misconstrued which could not be reproduced. This was the case with experiments related to tetanus, tuberculosis, smallpox, and diphtheria. Despite poor research protocols, support began to accumulate for additional research in the early twentieth century. Affluent families and industrial tycoons saw merit in the idea of creating a separate solution for each disease problem and benefitting from the profits.

By the time that the epidemic of so-called Spanish flu occurred in 1918, much of the world's population, including those who wrote the history books, had succumbed to the propaganda that germs were to blame. By World War II, few adversaries of the germ theory remained.

Over time, proponents of germ theory have adapted to the changing topography of discovery and research, rationalizing inconsistencies from the past with new findings, but continuing, as always, to claim the same thing, time and time again, which is that microbes cause diseases.

Germ theory is acutely dependent in most cases on a multitude of events occurring in conjunction. The probability of which, when analyzed, is so unlikely that even the most addicted gambler would not play those odds. To become infected by a microbe, first, a person would have to be exposed to enough of a germ to offset their health "defenses." Though scientists claim that hundreds of thousands of a bacteria can live on the tip of a pencil, it is also unlikely that these bacteria could live in such an inhospitable environment without nourishment for any significant period of time. They would need protection to survive long enough to be placed in the right location in someone's body for that person to be infected with them.

Time and again, scientists have tested samples of air, looking for microbes without finding adequate levels to "infect" an animal or human randomly.

Second, if enough of tiny "bugs" were located in one spot and did happen to become situated in a part of the body that it is possible to enter, then the conditions in this location would have to be suitable for sustaining, nourishing, and amplifying reproduction of the microorganisms. Additionally, the organisms would need to be able to ward off attacks from the first-line defenses of the infamous human "immune system."

As you can see, the odds of contagion causing illnesses requires a level of odds that is improbable. As a terrain doctor, I don't use words like *immunity* and *prevention* or accept that the body is under attack from microscopic organisms. Instead, I look at health as balanced or imbalanced and the microbes as synergistic components of the terrain.

The concept of contagion is dependent on ignoring other possible factors that might cause illnesses, such as environmental changes, toxins, malnutrition, physical misalignment, or even deep-seated trauma. If our government and corporations were to acknowledge alternate possibilities, it would threaten whole industries and the job security of numerous people.

By investing massive financial resources in health-care solutions built on germ theory and rationalizing the idea of random infection, our society has removed responsibility for our health from us and from our government and institutions. Years ago, tuberculosis and even smallpox were not seen as contagious, being that many lived unscathed alongside those that suffered from these illnesses. I contend that it was the popularization of the germ/contagion theory that turned them into contagious diseases.

The benefit of germ theory for the science of medicine-turned-into-an-industry is that it has helped standardize care and elevated the social status of people who promote it. It has also diminished the standing and reputation of those who oppose this idea, like midwives and naturopaths. Antimicrobials, vaccines, and other medications removed responsibility for doctors to dig deeper into patients' ailments and find the actual causes of their problems.

The textbooks used by history classes throughout our nation's grade schools typically cite germ theory as a breakthrough in medicine and an immediate triumph, but their authors are relying on biased sources of information. Other historical references don't share the same biases and show quite the opposite: that germ theory is unproven. Those who know the fallibility of the research still welcome traditional and natural medical approaches.

The industrialized culture's celebration of germ theory has weakened our belief in natural therapies, such as hydrotherapy, heliotherapy, and fasting, and created support for the synthetic pharmaceutical treatments that conventional medicine offers us, no matter how toxic. What immediately comes to mind is the dangerous chemicals used to treat people experiencing cancer.

Instant answers and one-size-fits-all Band-Aid solutions may seem gratifying. But what if individual approaches, like addressing our nutritional needs, receiving craniosacral therapy, sitting in the sun, and performing specific exercises, are more effective in the long-term?

Ever since germ theory came into vogue, we have constantly been told that we are organic "machines" and our health can be maintained through achieving sterility and uniformity of care. Whenever we meet a microbe, we are supposed to fight against it. We are therefore in constant battle to avert contamination and conquering by our "invaders."

Although promotion of bodily sterility has somewhat gone by the wayside in the last couple of decades, since we are surrounded by magazines and nutritional authorities who keep talking about our microbiomes and the natural microflora in our guts, there is still a predominant concern in our culture about catching diseases from foreign organisms. But some thought leaders in the conventional world of biology, like evolutionary biologist Paul W. Ewald, Ph.D., do believe that many of the organisms that have been linked to diseases are already harbored inside of us.

Although he may believe that almost all diseases are due to the activity of microbes, he does believe the body to be host to both "good" and "bad" organisms, living in a delicate balance. As Ewald writes, "Perhaps the experts are looking in the wrong place. Perhaps the most menacing infectious adversaries are already here."[1]

But are they adversaries? I don't think so. I agree with the eminent twentieth-century naturopath Stanford Kingsley Claunch, who pointed out that "germs are ubiquitous; they are everywhere, inside and outside of our bodies at all times, sick or well. The truth of this assertion cannot be gainsaid; consequently, it is impossible for germs to be the primary cause of disease. If they were, it would be impossible for us to be well at all because they are in us all the time."[2]

The Body Is not a Machine

The germ theory fits nicely into the idea that humans are machines—meaning that you can cut out a part when it is failing, halt a process by using some sort of medication, and ward off infections simply by creating barriers against them. But this belies the self-evident fact that our behavior over many years and the stresses our bodies endure contribute to poor health.

The body is not a machine, yet medical professionals specializing in the treatment of different body parts (hearts, lungs, kidneys, colons, and so forth) act as though organs in our bodies function separately and do not impact one another. Medicine sells the idea that we can remove an old, dysfunctional organ and put in a newer, healthier replacement without digging into how the original organ failed in the first place. There is flagrant disregard for the dysfunction of and weakness of the entire body.

People have become dependent on a system that can "fix" their machine and swap out their parts. Too little emphasis is placed on prevention strategies, like adjusting nutritional intake, and what else needs to be done or "put into the machine" to keep all its parts running smoothly and efficiently.

The *mechanistic view of the body*, which is based upon René Descartes's philosophical concept of *l'homme machine*, which says we are merely automatons created by God.

The institutional medical system has created specialist for each body part. The idea is that we are machines, like cars, that need tune-ups periodically. Each part is supposedly isolated so that if one is breaking down, you don't have to worry about it affecting the other parts. The body is assumed to run like a clock, which is not having trouble if its parts function within certain parameters; although it is not as integrated as a clock, being that a clock's gears are dependent on one another.

Science has always tried to simplify, identify, and label what it observes. Studies are designed primarily to answer the question of "why" things are happening, completely, so a simple remedy can be given—usually a pill or a surgical intervention. The machine view of calling a medical "mechanic" to "tune up" the body is a much easier belief to digest when it comes to our health than the view that we need to do better. It removes the responsibility of us being the "owner" of the malfunctioning machine and that there is a symbiosis within us.

Modern medicine reinforces the sense that we are not responsible for outcomes by teaching us to blame our genes, a stroke of bad luck, or the aging process. The machine has failed, not due to our misdeeds, but because something outside our control has "attacked" or "invaded" us, or a condition has developed in our bodies without our complicity or permission. This monkey wrench in the gears outlook is all too pervasive and has corrupted the deeper insights we could procure on the underpinnings of various ailments.

Genetics has long been a favorite scapegoat for developments in the body that seem extraordinary. But the fairly new science of epigenetics is teaching us to take back the reins of our health that we relinquished to random fate. *Epigenetics* is the study of how we can change the expression of genes in our bodies through modifications in our internal and external environments. Are we capable of switching on or off physiological processes by exercising, meditating, and eating in certain ways? Do environmental factors like polluted air and water impact us?

Other categories of study that are trying to address some of the mysteries of the health of the body are sociology and anthropology. These areas of investigation offer different aspects that, many times, regular biology neglects. The aspects studied in these fields show that an upbringing in a specific region, a person's gender, age, ethnicity, or even religion can color the viewpoint of a disease and its progression.

Even with rigorous experimentation, science has limited itself by going down a narrow road with gene theory. This theory does not resolve our lack of understanding about the dynamic interrelationships of our bodily systems and the functionality of all these parts within the whole. This is most apparent with the body's creations and reactions to illness and science's skewed explanation of the phenomena.

The germ theory became a dominant paradigm that allowed scientists to set aside any other type of experiment, idea, or belief that could make us aware of its inconsistencies or trigger questioning, even by experienced researchers. Science naturally tends to apply ideas in a linear way. Divergent ideas are looked upon as aberrant rather than a possibility of a new avenue of truth. We build on what we know or sometimes rather what we are comfortable in understanding. This has a negative effect on discovery and exploration. What we don't know, what we fail to explore because its aberrant, inadvertently is suppressed; knowledge that could potentially either complete the initial findings or discredit it all together.

It's important that we look at these earlier discoveries of old as a guiding light rather than crazy old men in need of accolades. Many of our current scientific beliefs are built upon the foundations of antiquity, so it is important to not throw the baby out with the bath water.

Traditional Cultures Knew Better Than We Do

The study of cultures, both living and dead, cannot be a neglected fact of this type of understanding: learning to thoroughly appreciate how the body works, especially in regards to health and the formation of disease through the lens of antiquity. It can give us a better appreciation of how health was seen prior to the germ theory indoctrination.

Although in most western and highly industrialized societies the body is thought to function like a machine, just responding to inputs, to this day there are still cultures which have not adopted this thinking. A few understand the importance of creating balance inside and out for their overall well-being, for themselves and their community.

For instance, traditional Korean medicine, *Koryo medicine*, which, like many other forms of traditional Asian medicine, dates back 3,000 or more years, sees the body as "part of nature and the cosmos, but one that is its own microcosm that constantly interacts with nature. . . . Practitioners of Korean traditional medicine say the ultimate cause of disease is not so much the intrusion of external elements, but malfunctions in inherent bodily function . . . Even diseases that appear to have external causes are ultimately seen as the products of internal factors."[3]

Western germ theory views every cell and organ in the body as separate and compartmented from every other cell and organ, and also sees the human body as separate and compartmented from nature. The people of traditional cultures do not relate to the world around them as if this is the case.

Indigenous cultures typically liken the body to an internal universe reflective of their outside world. They know that the body has dimensions that go beyond what can be measured. Those adhering to these traditions will call upon the wisdom of a shaman, medicine person, or folk healer to explain an imbalance in their bodies in terms of life events.

Illness is put in the context of a misgiving, poor hygiene, disharmony within the family, violation of a social taboo, or something supernatural that has occurred in response to misbehavior.

This wisdom, which has been handed down for generations through oral lore and only in the past several decades has been, and is now, being recorded in writing for posterity, honors the complexity of existence within the context of simple living. Whatever narrative is provided relates the illness to the negligence of the person or their environment.

Like ancient and indigenous healers, as a terrain doctor I contend that all beings we find inside and outside the human body, including bacteria, fungi, and other organisms, should, in fact, be approached as part of the whole, broad picture of the body and its wellbeing, and seen in the way that traditional cultures would see them: as synergistic components, mutually necessary for the maintenance of life and vitality.

THREE

THE NEGLECTED TERRAIN MODEL OF HEALTH AND HEALING

"The terrain is the physical manifestation of the body, the surrounding environment, and the etheric, astral, and spirit bodies. We view the state of the terrain in our emotional and physical reactions. In a very real sense, terrain encompasses the entire universe."

HARVEY BIGELSEN, M.D.

In the terrain model, it is understood that health and healing are determined by how well we nourish our bodies and support their functions. The philosophy recognizes that toxic substances (whether human made or naturally occurring) and a lack of their excretion, or trauma, with a loss of a balanced system, are the primary causes of disease. For thousands of years, this was the central belief to which every culture adhered.

In the late nineteenth and early twentieth centuries, many intelligent people fought against the idea of "germ" contagion as a source of disease, but their efforts were largely erased from the historical record by the propaganda of powerful drug companies and advertisers who amplified the idea with marketing campaigns created to promote their sales of chemical medicines. Then, in the late twentieth century and early twenty-first century a reinvigorated movement emerged that challenged the use of vaccines, questioned the germ theory and pursued more research in understanding the internal and external microbiome. The purpose of this chapter is to reveal forgotten and suppressed scientific knowledge to open your mind and introduce you to this way of thinking.

Here I will describe crucial studies done by scientists like Claude Bernard (a Frenchman who defined the *interior milieu*, aka *terrain)*, Antoine Béchamp (who discovered pleomorphism), Florence Nightingale (an influential nineteenth-century proponent of good hygiene and sanitation renowned for her service to soldiers on the battlefields in the Crimean War), among others who provided integral pieces to the puzzle of creating optimal health by respecting the terrain.

I will also refer to the recent work of modern champions of the terrain model, who include individuals such as the following three experts and researchers. Medical doctor and homeopath Hans-Heinrich Reckweg, M.D., who, in 1955, established the field of homotoxicology, the study of homotoxins (noxious substances) and the levels at which the body can successfully remove them or manifests disease from their influence. Holistic health pioneer and writer Sally Fallon Morell, who founded the Weston A. Price Foundation, a charitable organization "dedicated to restoring nutrient-dense foods to the human diet through education, research and activism" according to the mission statement published on its website.[1] Physician Harvey Bigelsen, M.D., whose dear friend cardiologist Robert Atkins, M.D., lovingly called him a professor of *terrainology*. Bigelsen devised a brilliant way of examining blood. All three are central figures in the field of new terrain medicine.

In terrain medicine, we understand that there are essentially four ways of regulating the body's terrain.

- Correcting the balance of fluids, nutrients, and structures in the body
- Supporting the microbiome to convert substances into something useful
- Eliminating anything that cannot be converted into something useful
- Eliminating excesses—whether from internal or external input—in every context you might imagine.

Metaphorically, the body is seen as a garden needing tending—a natural environment—by those who subscribe to this model of health care. Influences of contamination and mistreatment can change that garden, the germs only being the gardeners there to help clean up.

Where I Am Coming From

When I entered naturopathic medical school, I was acutely aware that its teachings would have little difference from those of the allopathic medical school I had just left. Studies of anatomy and physiology would be the same, and there would be little to no disparity in the explanation of how diseases manifest from genetic predispositions and exposure to bacteria and viruses. However, the naturopathic school would give me insights into the use of natural remedies and would emphasize the ideology of finding the root cause of people's health problems. It would encourage me to develop my comprehension of the whole body as an *integrated system.*

Where I was disappointed by my subsequent education was that when it came to resolving a disease, syndrome, or issue "naturopathically," the vast majority of the treatments I was taught to use were just greener and more natural alternatives to the synthesized pharmaceutical drugs that the allopathic medical school instructed students to dispense as well as "fight" and remove the germs causing the ailments.

During my training, I sought refuge in the written works of doctors who believed diseases arise from imbalances in the body as a whole. Because I mistrusted the approach of trying to "fix" an isolated symptom with a pill or reducing a holistic disease to a symptom-confined diagnosis, I separated myself from those who advocated compartmentalizing body parts. I particularly wanted to understand the body dynamic of all physiological processes working together in intelligent harmony. In the end, attending a naturopathic medical school confused me: The idea that the terrain, or inner environment, of the body could be healthy and balanced, but still susceptible to disease did not make sense. Why would the laws of nature allow for opportunistic microbial invaders to harm those of us who found a way to maintain optimal health? What would make a healthy person susceptible to germs?

Encountering inconsistency in my instruction, I dug in my heels and made a stand for the terrain model, the theory that the quality of our health is dependent on a multifactorial balance of the inner body and the outer environment—and to discard germ theory. My position as a student rep for a company that operated according to this belief afforded me the opportunity to solidify my knowledge about true holism, and follow in the footsteps of the predecessors of naturopathy.

The terrain of the body cannot be held together simply with a quick remedy or treatment. Despite this, many practitioners, including holistic ones, utilize natural methods in an attempt to achieve conventional, allopathic objectives. For example, if someone has a fever, that person is offered cool compresses. The root word *allo*, means "opposite" in Greek. *Allopathic* meaning a treatment is given in *opposition* to the symptoms being displayed by the body.

The findings of allopathic doctors and researchers always seem to point to microorganisms as the root causes of illness—belying the reality presented to them. For example, internal inflammation is a primary coping response from the body—healing and protective—to imbalances in the body's terrain, and known universally today as a strong causative factor for many degenerative diseases, especially when ignored. But in fact, microbes of all kinds work together with the body to respond to imbalances and clean up the mess. Environmental scientists witness bacteria's bioremediation constantly, yet when bacteria "bioremediate" situations in our own bodies, they're seen as the cause!

Let's talk about the alternate history of medicine now and some of the suppressed scientific data that back up the terrain model.

Claude Bernard (1813–1878)

Germ theory started taking hold outside of laboratories in the 1890s, when laypeople were introduced to it, but it was not broadly accepted and didn't start influencing public policy until World War I. While controversy about the nature of the connection between microbes and illnesses was underway, hardly anyone studied the impact of sanitation on health. Supporters of the terrain model (though it was not yet called by that name) advocated for better sanitation as a preventive measure that would help free sick patients from their symptoms. Good hygiene prevents people from being exposed to deleterious substances, like chemicals and dead tissue, especially when people are at their weakest.

Nineteenth-century French physiologist Claude Bernard was an influential scientist who formulated the concept of *la fixité du milieu interieur* ("the stability of the internal environment") as a significant factor in health. He observed that the body has mechanisms for dynamic equilibrium, and developed a list of factors he believed would elicit prevention from infections, which included[2]:

- Correcting the balance of fluids and nutrients.
- Converting something useless into something useful.
- Eliminating anything that cannot be converted into something useful.
- Eliminating excess.

The milieu of which Bernard was speaking is the French word for "environment of the body," internal and external, that naturopaths like me refer to as the *terrain*. I like this list and appreciate how people spoke plainly back then. They didn't know about vitamins and minerals or metabolic enzymes. But they did know that they ate food because it fueled their bodies. Conversion of something "useless" into something "useful" is a decent, plainspoken way of explaining digestion.

Take the digestion of a carrot, for instance. Holding a carrot in our hand makes it useless. But somehow when we chew and swallow the same carrot, the body turns this root vegetable into something most useful. We take that for granted today because we believe in carbohydrates, vitamins, minerals, and enzymes, and we know that the insoluble fiber will get pooped out.

Take notice that Bernard didn't put anything about eradicating germs on his list. Germs were not "on his radar." The thrust of his research was done to explain the body in physiological and chemical terms. As a result, he succeeded in making discoveries about the regulatory functions of the pancreas, liver, and vasomotor nerves.[3] Today it is common knowledge that the function of each of these organs supports the regulation of the terrain within us.

Bernard accepted that there are variations among individual people. Whereas Louis Pasteur's reports reinforced the idea that no matter the circumstances, germs will impact and invade members of a species—thereby concluding that a preventive measure, such as a vaccine, is equally needed by everyone—he would not have agreed with that. In his 1865 textbook, *Introduction to the Study of Experimental Medicine*, Bernard writes: "Physiologists and physicians must never forget that a living being is an organism with its own individuality."[4]

Like many of the most forward-thinking physicians of our own era, who recognize that our bodies are filled with what may be unique metabolizing neurotransmitters in the gastrointestinal tract, Bernard saw people's health as highly individual, and believed that neglecting to factor the uniqueness of their interior environments into treatment would lead to gross failures on the part of medicine.

Bernard was not a fan of the scientific establishment of his era. He patently believed that many scientists, Pasteur among them, were designing "experiments only to destroy a theory, instead of to seek the truth."[5] He openly expressed that so much vanity was present in the science of studying the body that observations and experiments were being skewed for the sake of gaining notoriety. And he said that once physiologists could see the body as a whole organism, they must consider the *harmony of this whole*, a foundational principle of the terrain model.

Bernard knew of Pasteur and Koch's research on "germs." While his expertise was not of identifying that our bodies contain trillions of symbiotic beings which are constantly aiding them in conducting routine functions, Bernard nonetheless believed that the presence of microbes in sick people was a consequence of an imbalance in their bodies, not the root cause of their condition. He insisted that stability of the body's inner workings is the basis for health.

When researching causes of disease, Louis Pasteur did not take quite a number of factors into account including environmental, so we can see that his research was flawed by the failures that Claude Bernard identified. During the nineteenth-century, industries such as hide tanning and cloth dyeing used public streams and small rivers for their activities. Families bathed in and drank from those waters, where toxic chemicals such as aluminum salts were washed off animal skins. Both people and animals also defecated in the streams. Water pollution is part of the external terrain that impacts our well-being since water is an integral part of bodies.

Florence Nightingale (1820–1910)

Nineteenth-century British nurse and social reformer Florence Nightingale was another proponent of the terrain model, though it was not formally known as such in her lifetime. She was a major proponent of cleanliness and sanitation, making sure many hospitals and medical institutions knew the importance of keeping their wards fresh and clean for the patients' sake.

Nightingale dedicated much of her life to the reform of the healthcare system of the British military as well as of the conditions for women during child birth. She served as a nurse on the frontlines of the Crimean War (1853–1856). Death rates were high among soldiers due to hospital-induced inflammation due to the reuse of muddied and bloodied wash rags, cots covered in urine and fecal material, heavy-laden air filled with soot and ash, and water that was sitting and polluted; which led to her conviction that the lack of sanitary practices was the cause. Later, she saw that the same applied to conditions and practices involved in delivering babies.

According to various reports I've read, Nightingale did not believe in diseases with specific identities. She also resisted the idea that disease could travel from person to person. She was convinced that symptoms resulted from poor environmental conditions, from the buildup of filth, putrefaction and decay in hospital wards, lack of exposure to clean air and sunlight, and fresh water to clean wounds, and clean sheets. Once environmental conditions were improved—which was accomplished without the use of the germicides and antimicrobial chemicals that are common in our society today—she saw the evidence of healing and health in the populations she served almost immediately.

Rudolf Virchow (1821–1902)

Even Florence Nightingale's contemporary, the so-called father of pathology Rudolf Virchow, known for his commitment to social, health, and political reform, did not necessarily accept the germ theory. Like Florence Nightingale, he was acutely aware that filthy living conditions and lack of access to clean water and adequate food impacted people adversely, causing sickness. He frequented derelict locations and witnessed people suffering due to poverty and a lack of social support.

Virchow wanted to improve the public health care system because he believed poverty and lack of essentials such as a clean environment, sunlight, and fresh air, caused ailments. He believed that doctors were using the germ theory to generate business to get paid for the solutions and medications they sold. He understood, just as Claude Bernard did, the constant of the internal environment (later called *homeostasis)* was dependent on the external environment and its balance and that the terrain can be impaired by worsening states of the external environment. What we today call a *cell*, he called a *vital element*. He writes: "The vital element (the vital unit), can be determined by the influences that come from the outside, or other elements or parts of this same organism, or of a body that is completely foreign, to certain manifestations of activity(actions, reactions)."[6]

Virchow was a forward thinker and another big advocate of social reform that he even led the construction for the

Berlin sewer system, knowing the importance of a clean environment.

It had been common knowledge since the seventeenth century that exposure to dust, dirt, and chemicals, as well as physical strain, could make people ill. In *An Introduction to the History of Medicine*, Fielding Garrison describes how Bernardino Ramazzini "opened up an entirely new department of modern medicine, diseases, and hygiene of occupations" when his observations brought focus to "such conditions as mason's and miner's phthisis (pneumoconiosis), vertigo, and sciatica of potters, the eye troubles of gilders, printers, and other occupations."[7] Both Nightingale and Virchow—and everyone else—knew that our environment plays an important role in disease creation.

Many key players in the public health and health care fields supported educating people about the importance of the external environment to internal health. Everyone agreed that unsanitary conditions were breeding grounds for illness, just not the reason why cleanliness matters. While there were doctors promoting the use of chemicals to clean wounds to kill bacteria, terrain proponents campaigned for clean air, water, and food, and sanitary workplaces and homes. These individuals included naturopaths, hygiene advocates, midwives, nurses, osteopaths, Christian medical doctors, and even some allopaths.

The History We Missed in Science Class

Historically, if you look for the cause of any epidemic or concentration of sickness in a region of the world you will see that it was preceded by a multifactor change in the environment. Something either changed in the place where the sick people lived or the people became sick after arriving in an unfamiliar environment.

As our ancient forebearers switched from a nomadic lifestyle to settlement in villages, they were confronted with new forms of leadership and industry. Multitudes of indigenous people have been impacted by feudalism, colonization, and forced agriculturalism.

In Europe, this type of social structure took hold after the crusades. A vast number of people who were disenfranchised by wars sought the support and protection of strong leaders. As walled villages expanded into kingdoms, the denizens within the walls had to submit to eating whatever food was brought in being that they were not farmers themselves. Most of Europe was divided into kingdoms with respective surrounding farms, which placed heavy burdens on the small farms due to constant fluctuating politics of religion, war, and climate. Any time there was a change in food production or a drought or flooding that damaged the crops, the outcome was devastating to these dependent kingdoms. Food and climate disasters were both important factors in the propagation of diseases. The highly variable outer world affects homeostasis inside each person's body.

The smallpox epidemic in North America among the Native people occurred after European settlers arrived and threatened them. Malaria and ebola in Africa, polio in the United States and India, yellow fever during the building of the Panama Canal in Central America, and on and on—pick any massive incidence of illness and you will find that conditions of starvation, impoverishment, and general psychological sorrow are already present in the society where it is occurring.

From 1346–1352, the bubonic plague or "Black Death" was an epidemic of massive proportions on the continent of Europe. Millions of people died, while countless others suffered for weeks, if not months, from serious skin ailments, fever, and gastrointestinal issues. The ramifications of this plague were imparted by the massive decline of industry, health, and population of almost all of Europe. But little discussion is made in history textbooks of the Great Famine of 1315 that preceded the epidemic. Although there was a separation of thirty-one years between the famine and the commencement of the epidemic, the amount of decimation and loss that occurred in Europe due to the famine required almost a century of correction.

Many do not know the extent of destruction or neglect that impacted livestock, crops, and living conditions in all of Europe. But for almost one year, rain and inclement weather destroyed hectares of the wheat and other grains growing in the fields. As productions of grain and vegetables declined, so did the livestock. An estimated 80 percent of cattle, pigs, and fowl died, leaving little to no food for millions of people.

Many people died over the course of subsequent years, and for generations afterward, were left with almost nothing nutritious to develop their bodies in a healthy way. Truly the only people that survived were those that lived separate from the dependence of kingdoms and economic trade.

Decades of redevelopment, along with numerous small wars across borders and between factions, hastened the psychological and physiological devastation. Increased levels of consumption of alcoholic beverages, along with the consumption of nutrient-weak foods, caused rapid decay in the health of people located in the more concentrated villages and towns. And as more hungry people relocated themselves to these concentrated zones hoping to fair better—perhaps being persuaded by the kings and leaders of those areas that they would—the living conditions degraded even further. People crowded together were exposed to garbage, excrement, and complete destitution.

From this standpoint, the inevitable became possible—a horrible disease passed through half of the continent. Two types of reactions are reported to have occurred during this time. One expression of the disease involved fever and enlargement of many important lymph glands in the abdomen and neck, which was not an uncommon symptom as it was also called *French pox* or *lues venerea* ("venereal plague"). The other expression involved darkened pustules covering the entire body.

As a side note, it is interesting to me that these two reactions were seen at the time as one disease, the Black Death, and yet, by current medical standards, these expressions would be understood as symptoms of two completely different diseases.

Another fascinating point of information relates to the lack of symptoms or epidemiological spread to many of the people who lived in the far northern part of the European continent in remote villages. According to the very first edition of the *Encyclopedia Brittanica*, produced in 1771, the bubonic plague only occurred in locations of heat and moisture, and even then, not during the cold seasons. It was also observed that the symptoms only showed up in the obese, the poor, and the overly indulgent, and women and children with "phlegmatic" constitutions (such as those experiencing chronic sinus infections and lung ailments like asthma).

Mainstream contemporary understanding of historical plagues has always erroneously attributed the spread of disease to a pest of some sort, such as a rodent, a flea, or a tick, and not to any ecological or psychological changes that occurred prior to the outbreaks. But we can clearly see that animals living together—whether they are goats, cows, dogs, or cats—all consume shared foods, lick one another and sleep with one another, and yet identical symptoms do not spread through the whole herd the way it did to the poor in medieval Europe, unless the animals become malnourished, and the weather or environment was unseasonably hostile.

In the twentieth-century, dentist Weston A. Price, D.D.S., studied undeveloped cultures whose people thrived without dental infections or disease. In the process, he determined that pasteurization and the incorporation of industrialized-processed foods in their diets were catalysts to disrupted health. Once these types of foods were consumed, symptoms of illness would sweep through small villages and the people's offspring would develop poorly and be stunted in much of their physiology and neurology.

Price's findings thoroughly demonstrated that indigenous people around the world living traditionally are more robust than their industrialized counterparts. In many of the communities he visited, epidemics were nonexistent.

Smallpox was wildly sensationalized as contagious and deadly in the late nineteenth century. Most often, the person experiencing the sickness succumbed to a fever and blistering. Yet the death rate was rather low, recorded at less than 1.25 percent among the unvaccinated, and in some places sufferers escaped death altogether. The historical references to higher percentages of mortality were recorded by doctors in hospitals working with the worst cases (none discerning between vaccinated and unvaccinated people). Accounts from doctors outside these institutions were left out of the history books.

One such account, in an article entitled "Hygiene," references the current understanding in 1872. I took the liberty of updating the language within the brackets to remove social biases.

> *Small-pox is a disease which is unknown either among* [Nature and natural habits of animals and humans], *it follows the civilization of* [Europeans]. *As soon as Europeans began to trade with the Indians, they (the*

> *latter) died of small-pox in masses; thus showing that small-pox is not born with many or a result of consequence of Nature herself, but that it is developed with the civilization* [of the Europeans]. *In a word, small-pox is not a phenomenon found of developed in Nature's laboratory, like death, but a companion of the* [Europeans'] *habits and customs.*[8]

This account also explains how the liquid excreted by the prolific blister marks called "pox" on the body is produced by an imbalance of salts and proteins in the blood. It was known, at that time, that alcohol *frees* the body of its salts and that alcohol consumed in excess leads to these same specific symptoms.

> [The Native North Americans] *died of smallpox because they expelled their blood salts by the use of liquor (introduced by* [Europeans]*) in excess, without replenishing salt in due proportions. As soon as salt became scarce in Paris, smallpox made its appearance . . . It is well-known, however, that a drunkard always craves salt . . . It is also well-known that, in general, the poorer classes, among whom the smallpox usually makes its greatest ravages, use less salt than the [upper]classes.*[9]

In translating countless scrolls and books written in antiquity, many translators working between the seventeenth and nineteenth centuries, misinterpreted the nature of the diseases that were described, imagining them as diseases familiar to them, such as smallpox and chickenpox, which made the current diseases seem to be older than they were. For instance, descriptions of fevers with malaise and intestinal symptoms were routinely labeled "malaria," while a description of a child with fever and sores on the body was labeled "smallpox."[10]This gave most of their readers the false idea that many of the diseases of colonialism and industrialism had occurred prior to their present day.

Also conglomeration of symptoms were named one type of disease in the past and historical accounts and renamed something different later on. This could also create confusion and misunderstanding to the lifespan, intensity, and severity of a disease and its supposed spread. An example of this is impetigo, a simple skin eruption, which according to the 1771 edition of the *Encyclopedia Britannica* was called "leprosy of the Greeks."[11] Leprosy, from our current understanding of it, sounds ominous to most people.

Without proper context, an epidemic or disease can be misinterpreted and mistakenly integrated into a historical narrative forever. With a better disease history, the number of causalities from a particular disease cluster can be analyzed more clearly.

Another nineteenth-century epidemic was cholera. Writing afterward, Max von Pettenkofer was able to illustrate how groundwater from porous rock mixed with air of a certain type gave way to people being affected by cholera. Places that did not have a cholera outbreak were places located over impenetrable rock. He investigated the conditions in various localities and was able to show that there were vast differences in the behavior of cholera regionally which could be uniformly explained. He satisfactorily explained the occurrence of cholera in some towns at particular times, and accounted for the immunity enjoyed by the surrounding people.[12] He writes: "As it is the result of a poison which springs from the soil, it is in this sense a miasmatic disease, just as much as marsh-fever."[13]

As you may recall from Chapter 1, early doctors often attributed symptoms to so-called *miasms*, antagonistic forces or "bad airs" underlying a range of conditions.

Pettenkofer believed the combination of carbonic acid with the air caused people to become sick. He also confirmed with several analyses that cholera was not contagious.

> *Cholera is not contagious, in the ordinary acceptation of the term, is established beyond a doubt by authentic circumstances such as the following. A ship put to sea with a detachment of troops on board, who have come from an infected town. A few days after embarkation Cholera breaks out among the soldiers, but not a single sailor takes it, although they are in constant attendance on them, and live in the closest contact. The disease, in fact, remains confined to those who came from the infected locality; and although their evacuations are exactly similar to those which on shore would produce frightful epidemics, the disease does not spread. Further, Cholera never occurs on shipboard unless introduced by persons coming from an infected locality.*[14]

He also emphasized how the excrement of cholera patients was not contagious when it was "fresh," but when mixed with water or sitting on the ground for some time was more of the problem, which meant it had to do with the ground or the water coming from the ground. During cholera outbreaks, Pettenkofer was able to deduce that many of the locations of the outbreaks were situated on wet, permeable land that caused the release of noxious gases. These gases are what caused the symptoms of cholera, not the microorganism found later. In his research, consideration was given to food and materials that were also exposed to the carbonic gases in or around the house and not cleaned, heated, or prepared properly as the cause of cholera in the household.

In an article in the March 1903 issue of the *Journal of the American Medical Association*, it was noted that there were no records of enslaved Africans having experienced tuberculosis, and despite the horrid conditions on the boats that carried them in shackles to the northern ports of America, they still did not "catch" tuberculosis as they traveled south from the northern ports where they disembarked the slave ships. The only occurrence of tuberculosis in enslaved people in the South, according to this article, occurred around 1830. The author claims it was confined to the "overcrowded and [un]sanitary conditions" in the Cincinnati slums and slums in other northern cities and was rare in the southern states.[15] The author attributes the difference to the quality of the water supply and the food they ate.

From before 1909 until about 1939, Flushing Meadow Park in Queens, New York, was nothing more than heaping piles of coal ashes. It was formerly known as the Corona Ash Dumps. This location was so famous that it was remarked on by a character in F. Scott Fitzgerald's book *The Great Gatsby*. The reason for its infamy was that the location was deplorable in standards of environment and safety. Marshes of the park contained life of various flora and fauna smothered in soot and destroyed by the mountains of ashes surrounding it and animal manure that was dumped there.[16] Many, if not all, the people of Queens and other surrounding locations were affected by the dark plumes of toxic ash that were swept up by even mild breezes.

This type of toxicity filled the air and it was not yet considered a source or even a contributing factor for the countless breathing, skin, lung, and even liver infections many of the citizens in the region complained of. But today, due to our familiarity with air pollution and different toxins, we can assume that tuberculosis, typhoid fever, pneumonia, asthma, and other ailments experienced by those people, logically can be attributed to its influence.

The so-called typhoid epidemic in New York State in the late 1890s was mistaken for a contagion. Before the advent of public sewage systems, fever was common throughout the United States. But the real reason was more likely that people were consuming toxic ice and using it to keep their foods fresh. One writer figured it out. In his 1891 book on water and ice, he says:

> *A considerable part of the ice supplied in ordinary seasons to New York and Brooklyn is cut on the Hudson River, and much of it just below Albany, where the stream is so greatly contaminated with the sewage of two large towns, Troy and Albany, as to be absolutely filthy. In both of these towns typhoid fever is of frequent occurrence during the period in which ice is forming. . . . There would, therefore, seem to be a very real danger in the use of some of the Hudson River ice.*[17]

There was absolutely no regulation of the removal of ice, and it was a thriving industry.

> *The ice companies, unless controlled by the State Health Department, will doubtless continue to cut and to furnish sewage ice along with the rest just as long as their customers will tolerate it . . . Ice-water is so cold that the nerves of taste are temporarily benumbed, and so the bad taste of much of the filthy ice goes unnoticed, and we are not warned.*[18]

Could it be that, quite possibly, upstream industrial toxins and excretions of toxic material were being ingested from the ice, causing people to become "sick" as their bodies were detoxing themselves?

One of the most infamous stories of the era was that of Typhoid Mary. This woman lived on Long Island in New York. Despite limited symptoms, she was incarcerated in city hospital because the authorities claimed she was the source of the spread of typhoid in the region. More than likely, however, getting the delivery of contaminated ice is what made people sick.

Another well-known epidemic was the Spanish flu of 1918. According to naturopath Benedict Lust, writing a year later, media reports of the day tended to inflate statistics about rates of mortality and hospitalization. And many people who received no particular treatment or used natural treatments recovered, while a "large proportion of cases [people] died under allopathic treatment."[19] His point was that though naturopathic care was better, the Spanish flu was merely something that could have been equally dealt with using simple measures, and it was not the highly infectious ailment one is led to believe.

In the United States alone, there were approximately 650,000 deaths from the Spanish flu. For those treated medically, whether with germ-killing medicines, aspirin, or other protocols, the mortality rate was 14 percent. For those that opted against any allopathic medical interventions such as these or utilized the age-old healing method of rest and chicken soup, the mortality rate was 0.9 percent.[20] When I look at these statistics, I cannot help thinking that in this instance the cause of death was certainly not a microbe so much as the treatments and the blind interference of allopathic doctors.

Elsewhere, Lust editorialized his own experience during that time when he was working in natural hospitals.

While our allopathic friends were futilely trying to check the "flu" with gauze masks, antiseptics, Dover's powders, and abundant food, and were wasting precious time trying to develop another poisonous serum from germs taken from the corpse of the "flu" victims, the Naturopaths were achieving unrivaled successes. The death rate from the pneumonia and influenza under Naturopathic treatment during the recent epidemic has been less than one percent. How does it compare with the 14–20 percent and even higher, under the allopathic treatment?[21]

What many do not know is that naturopaths and other natural doctors at the time did not use any products that killed or harmed the microbes in people's bodies that had been deemed infectious by the conventional medical doctors. This begs the question, how then did the patients survive the flu if the bacteria were not killed off?

FOUR

□□□□□□□□□

EARLY VIEWS OF MICROBES

"If a man loses his reverence for any part of life, he will lose his reverence for all of life."
ALBERT SCHWEITZER

Many medical practitioners in the early twentieth century believed that pharmaceutical drugs often caused more harm than they did good. Those traditional doctors were correct not to tamper with the body's intelligence, the self-balancing process known as *homeostasis.* But as industrialized medicine became big commerce and technology more sophisticated, the economy began to run on the success of corporate enterprises promoting chemicals. In this chapter, I would like to discuss with you that earlier, common-sense understanding of how the body responds to toxic poisons, the result of the action of toxins on the body, and how balancing actually occurs within the body. Big Pharma is a topic for a different chapter. Differentiation will be made between the mindsets of germ theory and the terrain model. Homeostasis and nutrition will be presented as complementary topics that help to explain what the terms *illness* and *disease* really mean in terms of what is happening in the body to maintain its balance.

What Causes Disease?

For a disease to manifest, specific conditions must be met. The root cause is never one simple trauma, one simple toxin, or one simple vitamin deficiency. Many factors have to interplay because we are complex organisms living in a complex environment. To simply say that one factor caused our symptoms is the reason we see confusion among scientists and laypeople alike. Take cigarette smoking for example. For sure, the heat and tar in smoke are toxins. Yet, not everyone who smokes develops lung cancer—or any cancer. Even sugar cannot be tacked down as the cause, despite being the notorious evil we are all taught it to be.

When toxins randomly enter the body (to distinguish them from substances we deliberately introduce through an IV drip, an injection, or anesthetic gas during surgery), the body needs to be at a lower than optimal level of imbalance for the effects of the toxin to cascade into creating the symptoms of major detoxification that our culture conventionally calls *disease*.

An example of imbalance in the body contributing to a detoxification event comes from an early twentieth-century outbreak of smallpox in Leicester, England. After vaccines were given to children by injection, several naturopaths and osteopaths—holistic health practitioners—recorded seeing all the symptoms of severe smallpox including death from it.[1] Public health officials wrote that despite the heavy vaccination attempt by officials, smallpox ravaged the town. As soon as the vaccines were stopped and sanitation improved, the smallpox all but disappeared.

Not taken into account were the living conditions that most of the children endured. They slept in filthy, over-crowded surroundings and ate nutritionally inadequate diets because their families were extremely poor. People in slums did not have access to fresh air, clean water, or sunlight. Many of these tenements involved in the outbreak were located near coal mining and processing plants, and many of the diseases the people's bodies expressed actually occurred following inoculations that were supposed to prevent them. All these components of the environment established the perfect conditions for severe detoxification symptoms to emerge, creating a widespread public health emergency.

This is not to say that the injections alone could have triggered the eruption of most of the symptoms in the population of the slums, but that without the low quality of their preexisting environment, their bodies could have metabolized and excreted the toxin better and they would have experienced fewer excruciating symptoms.

We need to address all influences on the human system to understand the totality of conditions affecting people's health, or else we mistake a natural process of physiological rebalancing for an infection by microorganisms.

What is a "cold," then, if not an immune response to infection by microscopic organisms? In terrain medicine, we view a cold as the body's attempt to cast out poisons and impurities in order to reestablish symbiosis and optimal regulation of movement of fluids and systems. Or as signs of an attempt to heal tissue that has been damaged in some manner.

Common colds are saving our physiological systems from falling into states of deep imbalance. Think of your next cold as a process of cleaning out your system, similar to cleaning house. Remove the junk and garbage and you will have space for things you need.

The symptoms of disease show up in two primary modes. Typically, they are:

- An attempt by the body to deal with toxic poisoning.
- A result of the action of toxins on the chemicals, cells, and tissues in the body.

But a combination of these two modes is also common. In any case, the body is responding by detoxifying.

Terrain Within

The terrain model believes that the health of the body is a constant ebb and flow of reactions induced by positive and negative conditions. With this model, it is understood that microbes play a primary role in the elimination of illness that we can perceive.

Although many health-care professionals do not know or won't acknowledge it, natural medicine is built on the foundational premise of the terrain model. Natural medicine encourages optimal health through adherence to a healthy lifestyle that includes choosing the foods we consume wisely, imbibing sufficient clean fluids, and sleeping, exercising, and socializing with likeminded people, among other things.

The difference between the terrain model and the germ theory is that the latter affords us the opportunity for complacency and to delegate responsibility outside us for every single morsel of food or exposure to a toxic substance. Germ theory has us worrying more about catching germs and less about bolstering and sustaining our physiological balance.

Living in an area where food crops are sprayed with pesticides or there is frequent consumption of processed foods can result in poor nutritional support for bodily functions. Giving rise to an imbalanced terrain, this causes a shift in the precursors (you remember, Antione Béchamp's *microzymas*),which adapt to forms that do the job of breaking down decaying material within the whole body. Those raised with the ideology of terrain medicine, who have been taught that every single item influences the "soil" in the "garden" of the body, realize how important their choices are in everyday life. All our choices positively or negatively impact our health. Every single thing we do, touch, apply to our skin and hair, and all the food that we eat affects the terrain of our bodies—the balance of their minerals, sugars, and all processes.

Pioneering French naturalist and biologist Jean-Baptiste Lamarck (1744–1829) believed transformation or any alteration in a species as a whole was the result of external influencing factors and the stimulus for adaptation on the individuals. Best known for his research on giraffes, he observed adaptive traits like the length of the neck being passed on to offspring, who could better reach leaves in high places. But it can be applied to any organism that replicates or procreates, including the microbes residing in our individual microbiomes.

In his book *Doctors Are More Dangerous Than Germs*, Dr. Harvey Bigelsen reports, "As the environment changes, biological organisms adapt, from humans all the way down to germs, and even one-celled organisms. Lamarck realized that evolutionary change is created by physiological needs."[2]

Many things affect the features that are responsible for how well or poorly the cells in our bodies function. The products we buy are made in bulk quantities in factories that emit plumes of toxins which can alter the terrain of the natural environment where we live. This also alters the characteristics of the microscopic inner world, like bacteria and fungi. In some cases, they adapt and become more efficient in their tasks of removing toxins.

Think about how bacteria have adapted to many of the antibiotic medicines our doctors have freely given their patients and become "resistant."

Being that we are mostly unaware of the adaptivity of the bacteria inside our bodies, as individuals we may be astonished when we *come down with a cold or sickness*, or a degenerative disease later on in life, after having been exposed to a chemical agent (even an antibiotic medication), at some point. But with the terrain model in mind, we understand that toxins have been building up in the bodily system reinforcing and furthering an imbalance. Finally, the body wants to correct this imbalance beginning by ridding itself of its accumulation of noxious materials.

In an article comparing naturopathy to conventional medical treatment published in the 1930s, Harold Detweiler writes:

> *The germ theory of disease was originated to explain the cause of disease and the transmission of it from one person to another. This theory was a life-saving element to the practice of medicine. It came at a time when the confidence of the people was seriously shaken and they were rapidly turning from Medicine to the other forms of treatment. This new theory was attractive, explanatory of many of the mysteries concerned in the study of disease, and above all, was highly technical. This technicality made it out of the question for the average layman to achieve any real knowledge of disease in general, or of the one he had in particular, and placed the power of cure directly in the hands of the Medical Physician. A germ was blamed for whatever the patient had and health depended on killing germs. Few people considered the fact that the same germs exist in healthy as well as unhealthy individuals. Science has been able to identify the specific germ as the causative factoring many of the diseases, in others no germ has been identified. It is well known fact that these germs exist whether they are producing diseases or not.*[3]

His point is correct. Given that sick and healthy people have the same microorganisms in their bodies, a different factor must be what makes one person express symptoms when the other does not. This is why natural medicine works far superiorly to conventional medicine when it is applied with the understanding of the homeostasis of the body and the importance of nurturing the internal terrain. If everybody were acutely aware of everything going on around them and took care with what substances they ingested along with applying the proper modalities that support the constant release of those toxins from the body, then we all could stave off the build up inside us that creates symptoms of sickness.

In an even earlier article, published in 1906, naturopathic physician Hans Knoch writes that what is called *disease* can actually be attributed to the health from within by which "large quantities of foreign substances are stored up in our body by breathing spoiled and used up air, wrong and unhealthy nourishment, which, besides nutritious parts, contains also poisonous substances, and by eating and drinking much more than is needed to replace the used up cells and to produce to preserve one's energy."[4]

Isn't it amazing that everyone used to know how important clean, unprocessed food, water, and air were to our health, and yet in the 120 years since Knoch wrote his article most of our society has forgotten this common knowledge?

The terrain model takes into account the idea that the inner body is an environment which will create the organisms it needs to handle the task of detoxification, like a well-run city where everyone is tasked with jobs to main efficiency and purpose. As opposed to thinking bacteria and fungi are malevolent entities causing disease, the terrain model views these microbes as beneficial symbiotic beings that support the body in forestalling further damage and destruction.

The exposure to toxins along with malnutrition are the key factors in disease manifestation recognized by the terrain model. Combined, these two things create a wonderful opportunity for deterioration in the body to occur on a grand scale, especially when the efficiency of removal by those very organisms is diminished.

While the terrain in which microbes appear is significant, the "germ" is not inconsequential. Terrain and microbes are interdependent. There is an important balance between the two when it comes to the creation of disease and the creation of health. Those are two different natural and complementary cycles occurring in the human body.

That said, when it comes to the body that is already symptomatic, the microbes that formerly were known as "germs," the bacteria and fungi that inhabit us, are crucial for removing toxic buildups of dead cells which result from traumas of sorts or secretions by our injured tissues. All kinds of byproducts are produced by the functions of the body. Hence, elimination is a natural, and ultimately necessary, process.

My point is that bacteria and fungi are not evil. They are very important in removing substances that must be removed in order to renew the balance in the body and support the terrain going back to homeostasis.

The earliest microscopes were invented in the seventeenth century. Since then, scientists have been studying microbes. Here are some of their reports.

In 1909, Hereward Carrington wrote:

> *I have long contended that, merely because germs were found to be present in certain disease, it by no means proved that they caused those diseases. The mere coincidence did not prove any casual agency no way or the other. In fact, there is a good deal to be said for the other side, that the diseased state caused the germ rather than the germ the diseased state.*[5]

In 1907, Ronald Campbell Macfie wrote:

> *These minute creatures, invisible to man for thousands of years, are yet the very basis and condition of his existence; for bacteria decompose dead organic matter, and elaborate nitrogen to form nitrates for plants. Without bacteria, there would be no decay, and decay is the jackal of life. Save for decay, dead matter would cumber the planet; save for decay, there would be no food for plants, and so no food for animals. Bacteria are the commissariat department of life. Suppose that suddenly every bacterium were killed. Then plants would perish from lack of food manufactured for them by the putrefying and nitrifying bacteria, and their seeds would be abortive. Herbivorous animals would accordingly starve, and carnivorous animals, including man, would die of famine. The dead would not decay, they would simply lie and dry*

on the last lichens of the exhausted soil, and the face of the earth would be like a museum or charnel-house with non-decaying leaves and flowers and with mummified corpses. For without the invisible cohorts of bacteria, the sun and the rain and the wind are impotent to evolve a single rose. Without bacteria, no flora, without flora, no fauna.[6]

Another doctor, Herbert Shelton, wrote in 1928:

The germs feed on the excretions. They are scavengers. They were never anything else and will never be anything else. They break up and consume the discharge from the tissues. This is the function ascribed to germs everywhere in nature outside the body and is their real and only function in disease. They are purifying and beneficial agents. The medical profession has worked itself into hysteria over the germ theory and is using it to exploit an all too credulous public. Germs are ubiquitous. They are in the air we breathe, the food we eat, the water we drink. We cannot escape them. We can destroy them only to a limited extent. It is folly to attempt to escape disease by attempting to destroy or escape germs. Once they are in the body, the physician has no means of destroying them that will not, at the same time, destroy the patient. We cannot avoid germs . . . We have to accept them as one of the joys of life.[7]

In 1921, George Starr White, M.D., wrote:

> *Nature never surrounded her children with enemies. It is the persons themselves that make disease possible in their own bodies. We must realize that one invaluable principle in Nature is* cause and effect *(karma), and every child should be taught that as soon as it is taught anything . . . Filling a healthy body with diseased matter to keep it well is so far from the natural way that it should have no place in the minds of intelligent beings. . . . Hygiene and proper living are the natural prevention of disease . . . We should all be taught that instead of germs being enemies and causing disease, they are friends and scavengers, and are attracted by disease.*[8]

Even way back then, there were two or possibly three schools of thought when it came to the terrain model way of thinking. The first, which is the belief I myself espouse, is that bacteria are adaptive and beneficial microbes. I do not believe they ever "flip" into being our enemies.

The second belief is that although the body can be healthy, any change in its status creates an opportunity for bacteria or fungi to invade, multiply, and cause damage. And by extension, that in a "sickly" (toxic) inner terrain, more opportunity exists for microbes to multiply exponentially.

A possible third opinion, which is an extension of the second one, is that some microorganisms *initially* help the body and *then* become hostile, if the environment of the body becomes too corrupted. For example, *E. coli*, a naturally occurring bacteria in our guts that benefits us by helping us break down our foods, suddenly become hostile.

In my opinion, people who believed that germs are hostile or pathogenic in any way, were sitting on the fence between germ theory and the terrain model. Today, there seems to be new interest in the nature of microbes within the context of the body. There is growing research on the gut biome and the skin biome, which you may be familiar with. For me, the first belief of our forebearers is borne out by the evidence. There is constant evidence of mutualistic symbiosis in the world around us, so why should our bodies be any different? A recent study shows over 1,000 different types of organisms living on the human skin, including 174 newly identified bacteria and twelve new genera of bacteria. These live in a state of balance on the body, all without harming the body or each other.[9]

Modern scientists are immersing themselves in research on the human microbiome, which is leading our culture away from a previously binary view of bacteria and fungi. Synthetic biologist Bernhard Päetzold, who works for a biotech company, for example, has stated: "The simplistic notion of 'good' and 'bad' microbes—a healthy or unhealthy microbiome—doesn't capture the true nature of microbial diversity and how it influences health and disease."[10] Although it is human nature to divide things into right and wrong, good and bad, friends and enemies, nature is not that way. Nature is holistic and unlabeled and everything in it influences everything else in the system.

Animals, plants, and insects are hugely dependent on the abilities of their microbiome, without which they would not be able to survive. In his book *I Contain Multitudes*, science journalist Ed Yong, whose research details the importance of all microorganisms and how every organism on the planet needs and benefits from their existence, states: "Microbes are not the enemies of animals, but the foundations upon which our animal kingdom is built."[11]

It is clear to me that only the terrain of the body (essentially, the body itself) changes, and that in no way do any of the microorganisms living inside it or on its surface—whether they're in the form of any type of microbe—contribute to the deterioration of healthy parts of the body. They are there to remove that which is undergoing decomposition.

Rather, when symptoms of sickness occurs, these are signs that the body's ability to remove a poison, toxin, or dead tissue in the terrain have become limited. Without limitation, the body would not fail to overcome a challenge, and symptoms would not arise.

Toxins and Ubiquitous Microorganisms

The more toxins your body contains, the more toxins will be liberated by the destruction of dead, decaying tissue, and the more bacteria or fungi are needed to take action to break them down. It's their natural job to handle the breakdown. They are *saprophytes*, organisms that eat only decaying material. Fungi are specialized saprophytes in that some can absorb many times it's weight in heavy metals.[12]

Fungi and bacteria are ubiquitous. In fact, they are the universally present organisms in our world. Without them, the soil would not replenish, and dead animals and plants would not decay. The first thing to show up in the disintegration cycle of life is the cleanup "crews" of bacteria and fungi.

Have you seen mushrooms grow on a fallen tree or maggots on a rotting animal carcass? These are the simple mechanisms of the cycle of decay. Because saprophytes are present in great quantity when there is tissue breakdown, we may deduce that their presence is indicative of cell death somewhere in the body.

To say that a germ causes the death of our cells when we feel sick would be akin to saying that the maggots (fly larvae) found emerging from the carcass of a dead deer in the forest caused the deer to die. How laughable! We know this not to be true, yet germ theorists think of bacteria and fungi as being harmful to our bodies.

Everywhere in nature, groups of saprophytic microorganisms living within diverse ecosystems clean up and create space for new life and growth to take place. They have an almost inconceivable power of multiplication when they are furnished with "food," nourishment from decaying or dead tissue. When finished with a "meal," which from our perspective is the task of removal of the nonfunctional tissue, they revert back to their primitive form.

In a coauthored book on germ research published in 1879, Louis Pasteur and Joseph Lister write: "We attempted the cultivation of the bacteria from an animal dead of septicemia [blood poisoning—author]. It is worth noting that all of our first experiments failed despite the variety of culture media we employed—urine, beer, yeast, water, meat water, etc. Our culture medium was not sterile, but we found most commonly a microscopic organism no relationship to the bacteria and presenting the form common enough elsewhere of chains of extremely minute spherical granules possessed of no virulence whatsoever."[13]

In Pasteur's own words, here is an example of the lack of contagion and the discovery of the precursor granules his adversary Antoine Béchamp named *microzymas*. We will talk more about them in the next chapter. The meaningful insight here is that Béchamp was able to disprove Pasteur's experimental findings time and again while validating his own results.

A measure of validity in science is how the same results can be obtained by anyone who repeats an experiment, as was done by Béchamp over and over again.

Pasteur also writes: "In many experiments I made on the blood in chicken cholera, I have frequently demonstrated that repeated cultures from droplets of blood do not show even development even when taken from the same organ, the heart, for example, at the moment when the parasite begins its existence in the blood which can easily be understood. Once even, it happened, that only three out of ten chickens died after inoculation with infectious blood in which the parasite had just begun to appear, the remaining seven showed no symptoms whatsoever."[14]

In his own words, Pasteur is saying he proved that something other than a transfer of a microbe caused illness, and that the supposedly diseased tissue did not always show evidence of the germ culprits as the cause.

I may be beating a dead horse (or chicken) here, but it bothers me a great deal when medicine ignores the immense impact of poor living conditions, lack of clean water, actual nutrient-rich food—as opposed to factory-made, nutritionless forgeries—and fresh air on our wellbeing. How is the body to build itself with food absent of nutritional value? It cannot, and so it eventually breaks down.

Even if we were to consider microbes "hostile," it is still evident from the research that there was a change in the terrain that preexisted their supposed hostility. This once again proves that the microbes are a secondary feature, in this regard, rather than a primary cause of ill health.

Microbes can produce substances (proteins) that break things down. This category of secretion is called an *exotoxin*. In my opinion, to look at these substances as *toxins* is a misnomer. However, that is the term used by mainstream scientists, so we will use it here, too. When an environment changes, the microbes begin their saprophytic activity.

For a long time, it was believed that a microbe's exotoxins were poisonous to other microbes and deleterious to the tissues of their human hosts. In fact, they seem just to be doing what they're supposed to be doing: expediting decay to make space for new growth. It is normal for the body to be eliminating cells that have reached the end of their lifespan or that were damaged or "manufactured" incorrectly. Bacteria can facilitate elimination.

Today, there remains a limited understanding of microbes and their relationship to disease; the same goes for the proteins they release. Researchers are investigating the microbiome and learning more all the time.

Endotoxins are fatty coatings (*lipoproteins)* on the surface of microbes that help protect them from extreme changes in their landscape. Complete information about this mechanism of protection has yet to be discovered. My reasoning is that this gives the bacteria time to adapt—to pleomorph.

To reiterate, my main point is that the word *toxin* is a misnomer. As part of their natural function to break down toxic substances, bacteria and fungi may produce endotoxins and/or exotoxins. Both types of excretion have been well documented in the context of laboratory experiments and within the bodies of humans and animals. What is not commonly known is the role that microbial "toxins" of both sorts play within our bodies.

Endotoxins and exotoxins may help activate elaborate mechanisms that otherwise would lay dormant in the body of a healthy person. These mechanisms may promote stronger detoxification along with the production of specific enzymes or chemical "markers" that teach the body how to respond the next time it is exposed to the toxin.

We could argue about how many ailments and inflammatory responses people experience due to endotoxins, yet the phenomenon of self-poisoning known as *endotoxemia* has only truly been observed within the last thirty years.[15] Short-sighted deduction can claim these microbial excretions as the culprit, yet when one takes a full view of humanity's level of exposure to pollution in the last thirty years alone, I can't help but think that those microorganic secretions are being used by our microflora to help strengthen their ability to break down toxic substances within us. They are doing human bioremediation, if you will.

Modern science has dabbled with the proposition that endotoxins are really exogenous hormones (*lipopoly-saccharides)*, and that neutralizing them is unnecessary. The truth is that they may benefit us, and they may harm us (though I don't think so), yet science still knows very little about what they actually do. It is an unproven matter that requires additional research.

To reduce the activity of saprophytes, one merely needs to support the body with the necessary components. For example, it has been proven that consuming vitamin C, such as in citrus fruits (the researchers used lemons), we can inhibit the presence of the diphtheria exotoxin.[16] This is simple evidence that gentle support of excretion can help rebalance the system without aggressive measures from the bacteria or fungus.

Lastly, when we see the abundant production of the bacteria in an illness and their excretions, regardless if one may believe in the terrain model or not, there still is a purpose for these organisms. The idea of invading germs is only a distraction to figuring out the real problem of the person who is sick. As Rudolf Steiner, founder of anthroposophical medicine, whose core principle is being in tune with nature, said in one of his lectures in 1920, "If only the natural history of germs were merely used as an aid to diagnosis, it would be extremely useful. You can tell a lot from the type of pathogen that is present because a certain type of microorganism always appears under the influence of specific primary causes."[17]

He made clear in another lecture that "you only need to be aware that the presence of [these microbes] shows that the person concerned has deeper-seated causes that allow the germs to accumulate . . . The actual organic causes lie in the human beings themselves."[18] Steiner was emphasizing the point that the presence of microbes in the blood and tissues of sick people is a symptom of a bigger underlying problem.

The constant findings of microbes during the ill state of health is compared to being guilty by association as Steiner stated in 1922 in a third lecture, " Those who claim that diseases come from small creatures, who say, for example, the flu comes from the flu bacillus *[a type of bacterium—author]* and so on, are of course just as clever as someone who says that the rain comes from frogs croaking. Of course, when the rain comes, the frogs croak, because they feel it, because they are in the water that is stimulated by what causes the rain. But the frogs do not bring the rain. Likewise, the germs do not bring the flu; but they are where the flu is, just as the frogs inexplicably come out when the rain comes."[19]

So, if germs are not bad, where, in fact, do they come from to do the work they do in our bodies?

FIVE

□□□□□□□□

THE KEY TO OPTIMAL HEALTH

"Microzymas are at the beginning and the end of all organized life."
JESSE MERCER GEHMAN, D.C., N.D.

At the naturopathic medical school I attended, microbiology was a required course, and one of our lab assignments for it was to do a project that would last the entire semester. Each student had to swab and culture the same object a multitude of times, after subjecting it to different media and environmental conditions. For my project, I decided to swab my cell phone.

As I made observations throughout the semester of the growths in my Petri dishes, I saw microscopic objects inside the cultured materials changing numerous times from round-shaped to rod-shaped and back again. Back then, I had a classical understanding of biology; I "knew" that microorganisms don't change form. Nonetheless, I observed what I observed and assumed I was witnessing something that was well-known to people at the graduate level of microbiological study. When I showed my notes about this phenomenon to my professor, he explained that I had to be mistaken because "organisms do not morph into one another."

I thought the discrepancy between what my professor told me and what I was observing was kind of odd, so I continued to culture my specimen. But as I submitted additional notes, which I felt were accurate, I kept getting poor grades because of the findings I reported. It was presumed that I had either a terrible swabbing method or a nonsterile culturing method, or that another factor was interfering with my results. The consequence was getting low marks because my specimens appeared to me to be changing despite several attempts to do what my professor suggested. I even spent extra hours in the lab so I could make additional observations.

After two more weeks, I asked the professor to help me swab my specimen again, redo the culture, and look under the microscope along with me. When he did, he observed the same changeable behavior as me, and said, "Well, I guess there is something very interesting and altogether strange going on here, so you just have to submit the results with a full explanation of your methods." At last, my lab work was not dismissed as incompetent. My grades went up.

Later, when I was introduced to the terrain model, I learned that what I had been watching was the phenomenon of *pleomorphism*, a term taken from the Greek roots *pleo* meaning "more" and *morphism* meaning "the state of being a shape." I had stumbled upon the hidden world of microbial precursors (aka *microzymas*). Doing this experiment is what led me to discover and be fascinated by a whole world of microbiology that, historically, has been suppressed, and it was a life-changing experience for me.

Precursors are where all microbes come from that scientists observe.

Conventional scientists do not agree with this assertion.

While Louis Pasteur was discovering supposedly causative agents for the diseases that surrounded him, various bacteria, fungi, and parasites, another scientist of his era, the man who was his chief rival, was conducting research that was proving something different. Pierre Antoine Béchamp, a French medical doctor and chemist of renown, demonstrated that germ theory—or as it was called at the time, *microbian theory*—had a shaky foundation.

You've already read what I think about germ theory, so in this chapter, I am going to explain what I believe is going on instead on the hidden, microscopic level of our existence.

What Béchamp discovered in reference to the body, disease, and health were "little bodies" (his description) that he named *microzymas*, from the Greek roots for "small" (*micro*) and "ferment" (*zyme*). He found these everywhere, including in both living and dead bodies, and believed them to be of great antiquity due to also finding them in rock strata that had been assessed as being millions of years old.

Béchamp's microzymian theory of living organization led to the discovery of a so-called *third anatomical element* in blood: the microzymas. He called them "living organisms of an unsuspecting category," and claimed, "The microzymian theory of living organization gives biology a base as solid as the Lavoisierian theory to chemistry…"[1] He was referencing Antoine-Laurent de Lavoisier's contributions to the field of chemistry during the eighteenth century, which it basically changed the course of chemistry forever.

If you were to look through the lens of a modern light microscope with a simple dark field condenser, you would personally be able to see microzymas in samples of blood. Working together with the body, microzymas organize and facilitate many, if not all, of the various processes of the body, including maintaining cellular vitality, supporting cardiovascular integrity, and promoting proper cellular replication.

Being that they function to maintain homeostasis on a cellular and subcellular level, we can view these microzymas as elemental units of colloid protein-based life. (This is why I use the term *precursor* for them in my own writing), although I'm under the impression they have minimal physical form, if any form at all, at a submicroscopic level. Basically, every cell and living organism needs these precursors to thrive and survive, and if you remove them from cells, the cells die.

Béchamp's Three Most Significant Discoveries

During his lifetime, Béchamp made three important discoveries about microzymas. The first is that microzymas are anatomical structures that supply all the cells in our bodies with the proper physiological and chemical environment for us to live in a perfect state of health.

Béchamp's second discovery was that when microzymas are removed from animal tissue, the tissue no longer functions normally and this leads to tissue disorganization. After a few days, cells eventually die and release their microzymas. (This release may be what many mistakenly think of as *viral shedding* as viewed through an electron microscope.) Many scientists in later times, who have studied microzymas, posited that what was thought to be viral particles, when they became more formally discovered by conventional science, were merely snapshots of the microzymas inside and outside of the cell. They came to this conclusion because of analogous location, behavior, and size.

The third significant discovery Béchamp made is that microzymas actually changed (aka *pleomorphed)* into various forms, including bacteria or fungi that surround cells under altered conditions. In these forms, they are capable of consuming dying and dead matter that used to be living tissue. The dead tissue is a different kind of *terrain*, or biological landscape, than living tissue. The indication of dead or decaying matter in the surrounding environment (terrain) of the cells calls to the transformation need of the microzymas, basically to change their job from support and maintenance to clean-up crew. As bacteria or fungi, microzymas will finish up their "food" and then change shape again, devolving themselves with the aid of other conditions, like detoxification, oxygenation, and a steady supply of nourishment to the terrain, until they may reassume their precursory microzymal state.

Béchamp did numerous valid and reliable experiments during his career using the microscopes available in his era to carefully observe how microzymas move through different stages and assume the forms of various bacteria. He was able to do this because he was able to isolate them and demonstrate their changes, repeatedly. Bechamp then repeated the identical experiments, using all the same materials *except for* the suspension containing the microzymas, and they never yielded the bacteria. There were many detractors to his work. Microbiologist Robert Koch, for example, believed that all the stages of microzymas that Béchamp catalogued actually are different species of bacteria, separate from one another, despite the fact that Koch and Ernst Almquist themselves observed various forms within the blood of people with typhoid symptoms.[2] Yet, Koch did not agree that pleomorphism was possible, only simplifying the reality of what he saw.

Contemporary naturopaths, such as me, who embrace the indications of pleomorphism, believe that microzymas are always attempting to maintain or reestablish harmony in the body. They are an integral part of our internal and external terrain. They are present in our blood and lymph, and in various internal organs, as well as on the surface of our skin.

Béchamp's experiments led him to understand that any bacteria or fungi found in or on our bodies have been "freed" from their normal state of existence. In time, they will revert back to their original, simple precursory form. In one of his most interesting experiments, a kitten was killed and buried between two beds of pure carbonate lime and left in a glass vessel so the corpse could be observed. A small quantity of paper was put in the glass vessel as well, so that air had free access to it, but dust was excluded from entering the vessel. It took seven years for the carcass of the kitten to completely disintegrate. Some fragments of bone were left at the end of this decomposition period, but the majority of the kitten disappeared. The carbonate of lime was white, and it was completely destroyed as well. The color of the lime indicated that no biological material remained. Under Béchamp's microscope, nothing was left in the glass vessel except for crystals and crowds of little granulations or spherical bodies, the microzymas.

From this experiment, we can conclude that these fundamental life forms are virtually imperishable, capable of surviving even the harshest conditions. Once all the living material around them disappears, they basically become crystalline dust.

The Benefits of Cellular Pleomorphism

In order for us to create optimal health, it is important to understand that the many microzymas that surround each and every cell in our bodies work diligently to maintain balance and health in our physical systems. Likewise, they clear the surrounding environment of debris, which they do by altering their appearance and functionality to become saprophytic bacteria or fungi. This pleomorphic transformation is necessary in order for the microzymas, in the form of saprophytes, to do the task of removing our bodily wastes to create a more hospitable environment for living tissue and their vital functions to occur.

If the environment of the human body is kept regulated and clean through ingesting proper nutrition, exposure to sunlight and clean air and water, sound sleep, and sufficiently few external stressors placing demands on its systems and processes, then the "little bodies" in our bodies, the microzymas, stay just like that—little and precursory. But if the terrain of the body is disharmonious, perhaps because it has been neglected, abused, overtaxed by stressors, malnourished, and/or encumbered with toxins or excessive levels of deteriorated tissue, the pleomorphic transformation occurs and the microzymas become the organisms needed to address the issue. They assume an appropriate shape for the activity that needs to occur in the specific location in the body, adapting to whatever has happened.

Béchamp set out to demonstrate that the microzymas were actually living beings and that they contributed to the life force of the organisms in whose interior they lived. So not only was he trying to prove they existed, but he also sought to prove that their existence was of an autonomous nature—meaning, not glandular secretions or fluids manufactured by our own bodies. In 1886, Pasteur admitted that he too had observed the presence of microzymas in blood. But he brushed them off as molecule granulations that may have contaminated the sample. Other scientists also brushed them off, identifying them as white grain, minerals, fat, albuminoids, and other items. Only Béchamp believed that the microzymas were disappearing and reappearing when needed. He noted microzymas in various mediums and understood that mass quantities were present in the body as well as in soil.

A race was on to identify underlying causes for disease. The bias that began in science was to view microbes as foreign invaders and enemies out to damage the body's resources, rather than as coresidents of the body and allies in creating optimal wellness.

One of Béchamp's nineteenth-century contemporaries, Casimir Davaine, was studying anthrax bacteria as a source of disease. He concluded that they were not. This study reinforced Béchamp's belief in microzymas. He commented: "The bacteroides were not the cause of the disease condition but were one of its effects; proceeding from the morbid microzymas they were capable of inducing this disease condition in the animal whose microzymas were in a condition to receive it. Hence it is seen that the alteration of natural animal matters is spontaneous and justifies the old aphorism so concisely expressed by Pidoux; 'diseases are born of us and in us.'"[3]

Pidoux was a doctor from the Middle Ages.

Pasteur was a chemist, not a physician or physiologist, and yet he pushed his germ theory and condemned microzymal theory quite feverishly. Even so, when Béchamp was in the French Academy of Medicine, none of his colleagues was able to prove him wrong. They were only able to associate a disease in their animal test subjects with a microbe *after* they removed the microbe from a sick animal when it was already displaying symptoms, and not before—essentially committing what's called a *confirmation bias*. In other words, *after* pleomorphism had occurred.

It has been postulated that microzymas last forever, that they cannot be destroyed. They live everywhere in the environment around us, and they also live within us. Once a body dies and decays, the precursors in it go back into the soil, where they live on. Bacteria are ever present in the soil, the reason they are there is to assist in the process of decay. Once this process is done, they will revert to their pre-cursory state.

We could say that health is a well-managed terrain in which the microzymas successfully break down all unnecessary material while the body efficiently excretes all that is toxic and damaging.

Some naturopaths view the work of the microzymas and their pleomorphic capabilities as a separate issue than the issue of healthy terrain, yet this explanation of the source of bacteria and fungi is actually, for me, an integral consideration when planning how to help a patient or support our own detoxification and healing functions.

It is widely accepted that bacteria are not stagnant; they do not hold one, immutable form, as Louis Pasteur believed they did back in the nineteenth century. The principle proponents of pleomorphism early on were Drs. Ernst Almquist, H. Bergstrand, E.C. Hort, F. Lohnis, P.F. Clarke, Edward C. Rosenow, and Günther Enderlein. Later there was Royal Rife and even more recently, Drs. Maria M. Bleker and Harvey Bigelsen.

After the Spanish flu, H.W. Wade and C. Manalang discovered that the bacteria which, during the time, were thought to have caused the influenza, would occasionally abandon their common form and become more fungus-like, along with producing spores.[4]

Today, everybody knows and accepts that a coccus (circular-shaped) bacterium, doesn't stay in a circular form in every single environment to which it's exposed. It changes into other shapes when environmental conditions are altered, like a rise in pH, or the presence of blood where there shouldn't be. But when Wade and Manalang's report was published, there was constant and obvious criticism of their belief in pleomorphism (as there still is). The scientists were attacked for having poor technique, for possibly contaminating their samples or manipulating or misinterpreting the data. Later, as some of their critics conducted similar experiments, the critics were unable to dismiss pleomorphism as the cause for many of the changes they were seeing with their own eyes.[5]

The Research of Zoologist Günther Enderlein

Apart from Béchamp, a multitude of scientists, such as immunologists and microbiologists, have done extensive studies that show bacteria present in all types of tissue, and how these microorganisms mutate in form when exposed to different environments and different tissues. The earliest of these researchers was Günther Enderlein, Ph.D. (1872-1968), a renowned zoologist who discovered and named many insects, went on to witness tiny granular bits in the blood working in a peculiar manner with the bacteria in 1916 when he was studying the blood of soldiers in WWI.[6] He came to the same conclusion about the reason the tiny granulations were present that Béchamp did: They were working to promote decomposition from the body.

Isn't it interesting how the belief systems and biases of scientists affect their findings? Remember my professor of microbiology grading me poorly despite my observations being accurate? Perhaps because he was less mentally rigid, Enderlein was able to witness the changing of the forms more readily than other scientists of his day who conformed to the belief that microbes can never change form. Because of his unbiased observations, he succeeded in measuring the various stages that microzymas cycle through, and developed a template for these mutations that he called *bacterial cyclogeny* (see figure 5.1 on the next page).

When looking at the illustration, notice how the most primitive forms are situated at the beginning of the cycle, and the more complex fungal forms at the end of the cycle. The bacterial forms are intermediate phases of transformation.

Based on this template, Enderlein was able to identify multiple lifecycles for bacteria, and also discovered a type of nucleus inside of them that is different from the nucleus of cells found in humans.

Rather than call the form in its granular resting phase that Enderlein observed in these microorganisms a *microzyma*, the way Béchamp did, Enderlein termed the form in that

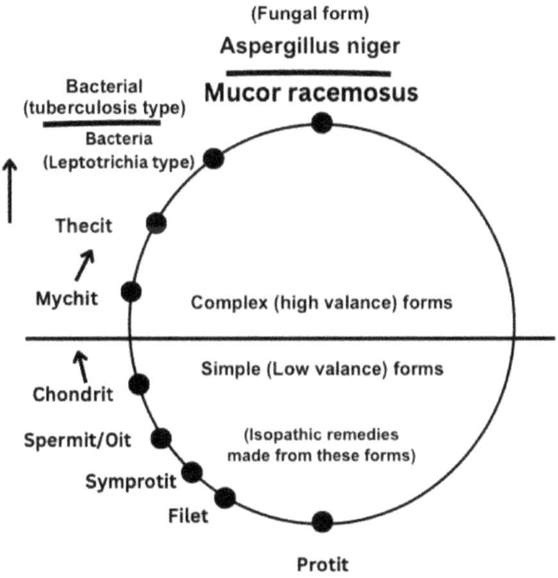

Figure 5.1 The Enderlein cycle of bacterial pleomorophism.

precursory phase a *protit*. In discovering the changes of which they were capable, he ascertained how tiny protits develop into more complex forms depending on the nature of the environment around them, even under their most minute changes. A granulation adapts from its resting form into a bacterium, then into a fungus—a stronger form of saprophyte—if the terrain around it begins to deteriorate more extensively or if the tissue does not offer a good environment for the bacterial form to thrive. And it is during more advanced states that replication and reproduction occur because abundance is needed to clean the body more efficiently.

To reiterate my earlier point about microzymal adaptations occurring in order to maintain the balance of the body's internal terrain, please remember that the main reason microgranulations (or precursors) advance in their lifecycle and transform into bacteria is because something in the terrain—the body's homeostasis—has changed. This change could be in the level of what is perceived as hormones, organic acids, cellular excretions, a release of protein substrates due to tissue breakdown from dying cells, or a decrease in nutrient status, and so on.

Enderlein believed that the pH of the body and blood play an important role in the transformation of the precursory granulations. He intensely focused on studying the activity of the precursors situated in different locations of the body, trying to determine how they were working to facilitate and support the activity of that particular tissue. How they would help a brain cell and how they would help a liver cell, for instance, would differ. Believing some protits to be "primordial symbionts," that have been passed down generation upon generation *in utero*, he named them *endobionts*.

According to Enderlein, a catalog of two types of endobionts maintain the homeostasis of the body's systems: *Mucor*, a fungus in its culminate stage, maintains circulation. *Aspergillum*, another fungus in its culminate stage, maintains muscle, skeleton, and skin.[7]

Here's an example to give you a better understanding of how the precursors work. Let's say you go for a jog wearing very tight running shoes and you've been feeling under the weather. Due to having some sort of preexisting deficiency in your terrain, your feet are damaged during your run. Now, the endobionts in your feet transform into derivatives of the aspergillus fungus to clean up some destroyed tissue. Today, we would say that you have a case of acquired toenail fungus because you didn't wash your socks or your shoes were damp. But in truth, you did not replenish your body with the proper nutrients before or after the run; nor did you maintain adequate oxygenation during the run by means of proper circulation. The endobionts in your feet are there to help maintain their respective tissue, just as they do in other locations throughout your body, and the fact of the matter is that they are doing their job, as Enderlein proved a multitude of times—in this case, by transforming themselves into saprophytic fungi in your toes.

A more current theory, which not only supports Enderlein's discovery of protits, but the origins of pleomorphism itself, is the *serial endosymbiosis theory* (SET) of the origin of cells, about which the late evolutionary biologist Lynn Margulis wrote extensively. She theorized, through her observation of the world around us, that all *eukaryotic* cells—a category of cells belonging to complex organisms like animals, plants, and fungi—evolved from the fusion of simpler organisms, including various bacteria, molds, algae, among other things. In this way, each organism contributed in a specialized function within the merged community, making them highly dependent on one another.[8] We see this very idea reinforced by the speculation of many microbiologists belief that the mitochondria, the powerhouse of our cells, are probably descendants of bacteria that symbiotically implanted themselves within our cells long ago.

Now, if bacteria with a specific function are constantly formed within our cells, the possibility of pleomorphic development of organisms is not so farfetched, especially if they are first starting within our body in a less complex form. Writing fifty years prior to Margulis, Enderlein asserted the very same thing regarding the specific form of the precursors known as endobionts. These are the ones that he believed to be passed generation to generation through the egg and sperm.

What modern science calls *immune cells* are simply these endobionts doing their jobs. Perhaps instead of genetics, we may have to look into the inheritance of these precursors and their behavior as what is "passed down" rather genes and genetic "tendencies"

The Research of Biologist and Naturopathic Doctor Gaston Naessens

French-born biologist and naturopathic doctor Gaston Naessens, N.D. (1924–2018). discovered the same things that Béchamp and Enderlein had found in their research—precursors of bacteria circulating in the blood of humans and animals, and sap of plants—and called them *somatids*. He was able to see these ultramicroscopic living particles through the lenses of a special light microscope he designed, the somatoscope, and to catalog their pleomorphic cycles. Naessens identified these somatids as indestructible lifeforms within our bodies that may have lived thousands, if not millions, of years, reproducing and being handed down generation upon generation from our ancestors to us. Similar to the tardigrade (aka water bear), the somatids were shown to be virtually indestructible by surviving exposure to carbonization temperatures of 200 degrees Celsius and exposure to 50,000 rems of nuclear radiation.[9]

Through the somatoscope, Naessens has observed somatids morphing and displaying sixteen separate forms in stages that he terms the *somatic cycle.* He has captured images of these stages using stop-frame photography.

Naessens has been able to correlate disease states with respect to the *somatic cycle. Disequilibrium* of the body is what he concludes sets the somatids (or precursors) on their pleomorphic cycle. Knowing this, Naessens is able to predict the occurrence of a disease by looking at a person's blood prior to them exhibiting any strong outward symptoms. Over the years, as he did more and more research, he has come to view somatids as the "precursors of DNA."[10]

Interestingly, the measurements of the precursors within the initial stages of their pleomorphic cycle are generally tinier than the measurement of what is considered a virus. He was able to see precursors because the somatoscope does not destroy tissue samples the way an electron microscope does. One may ponder, quite possibly, if what mainstream scientists think of as a virus is simply somatids in an area of the body doing their detoxification work as nature intended.

Naessens believed that precursors give life and are called to act upon the cells by the body depending on which direction its homeostasis is going. He experimented with the actions of somatids by adding them to a piece of raw meat or a grafted piece of skin and witnessed growth of tissue in both cases. Neither tissue displayed rejection or what is considered in current scientific terms "infection."[11] As Béchamp discovered one hundred years ago, Naessens has confirmed that that germs are not the causes of disease but energized and electrical bedfellows that, in fact, help us restore our health. Germs are not our enemy.

The Research of Inventor Royal Rife

Another twentieth-century inventor who created a microscope just a few decades before Naessens also discovered the electrical nature of precursor micro-organisms. His name was Royal Rife (1888–1971). In 1913, he started his journey of learning about bacteria and of developing a microscope. By the late 1920s, he had completed a design for a microscope that was far more powerful than any other of his era. Using handmade, many quartz crystal lenses packed in glycerin, this microscope magnified objects by a factor of 17,000.

Microbiologists looking at cells under a microscope typically stain them with colored dyes to help them better visualize their components, such as the nucleus or the cell wall. Interested in investigating viruses, Rife invented a way to "stain" cells with a light frequency modulating machine instead of conventional chemical dyes so microorganisms would not be killed in the process. At the time, microparticles had been seen within cells, and many were assumed to be viruses because there was no way for scientists to clearly differentiate them from other particles or bacteria.

Being that Rife was equipped to see in his microscope the particle that his colleagues were calling a virus, a particle that was said to measure 1/15 to 1/20 of a micron, he ended up verifying the existence of the precursors and pleomorphism.[12] As he introduced particles into different mediums and watched them change forms under his microscope, Rife's findings confirmed similar findings from Béchamp, chemist Edward C. Kendall, Ph.D. (who won a Nobel Prize in Physiology in 1950 for studying adrenal hormones), Edward C. Rosenow I, M.D., head of experimental microbiology for the Mayo Foundation from 1915–1944, and other bacteriologists who had observed pleomorphism before him.

In doing research on microbes, Rife only sought to understand the causes of disease. Because of his discovery, however, Rife stated:

> *In reality, it is not bacteria themselves that produce the disease, but the chemical constituents of these micro-organisms enacting upon the unbalanced cell metabolism of the human body. . . . We also believe if the metabolism of the human body is perfectly in balance or poised, it is susceptible to no disease.*[13]

The Research of Wilhelm Reich, M.D.

Psychoanalyst, scientist and apprentice under Sigmund Freud, Wilhelm Reich, M.D. (1897–1957), who was the developer of the techniques known today as the system of bioenergetics, was a visionary who was heavily censored in the United States for his interest in biological energy, which he called *orgone.* His writings reveal that he knew the importance of the little precursory specks found in living things and nonliving objects alike, calling these precursors *bions,* and did not believe they were culprits in creating disease.

In his second volume on orgone, *The Cancer Biopathy,* published in 1948, Reich repeatedly demonstrated the absurdity of germs being transient in the air to contaminate and infect larger organisms. He viewed the lack of acknowledgment by medical researchers to accept that organisms were constantly being furnished within living beings as an obstacle to correct treatment of disease.

> *Not only is the air-germ theory false and incapable of providing enlightenment about the central phenomena of biology and pathology; it actually hinders a factual comprehension of the mechanism of disease. It has become a dogma which, like all dogmas, eschews thinking and inquiry.*[14]

Reich looked at the bions under a microscope and saw them glowing, so he postulated that they contained the energy he called *orgone,* that initiated biological effects in cellular structures to either promote their health or to expedite movement and cellular breakdown. He believed orgone flowed through everything in existence. He also believed that energy is the factor in the body that creates health. He stated that orgone helps tissue regenerate and gives vitality to the soil in which plants grow. Reich's theories align with the principles of traditional Chinese medicine and ayurveda, which recognize energy channels in the body. But the American government was not open to anyone even discussing these concepts.

What is fascinating to me is that yet another scientist discovered the primitive, yet hyperintelligent precursors to microscopic living structures. Bions are one and the same as Béchamp's microzymas, Enderlein's protits, and Naessens' somatids. These microorganisms, or energy creators, if we concur with Reich, create a network in the body through which the life force flows that helps us maintain our internal processes and thrive. Every cell, every living thing, is able to function properly with it.

The Primo-Vasculature System and the Theory of Sanal

In the mid-twentieth century, surgeon Bong-han Kim, M.D., who defected from North Korea, discovered a network within the human body, the *primo-vasculature system*, which corresponds to the meridian lines used by acupuncturists to modulate the flow of life force energy. More accurately, this system is the "circulatory network system where microparticles interact to form and breakdown cell structures in response to biological conditions at the subcellular level."[15] The term he coined for these particles, which are precursors, is *sanals.*

After Kim was provided an institute by the government of South Korea to further his discovery of the sanals and this network, he was able to identify and anatomically map out, using dyes and contrast agents, many of the channels, ducts, and ductules through which sanals travel within the body. Many of them are located within capillaries and lymph vessels.[16] (See figure 5.2 below.)

Kim also examined the behavior of the precursors, and confirmed the analysis of both Bechamp and Enderlein, which is that precursors interact with one another, form larger particles, and eventually become cells.[17]

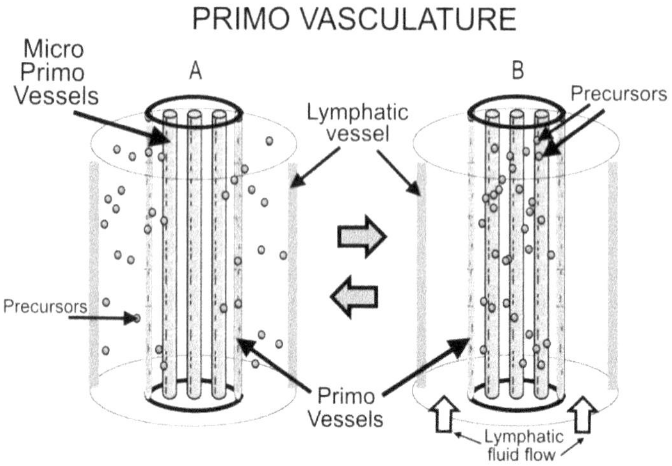

Figure 5.2 The primo-vascular system.

Thus far, despite the strong evidence Kim presented for the existence of another vascular system within the mammalian body, minimal effort has been made by mainstream researchers to explore the extreme importance of his findings.

More Researchers, More Nicknames for the Same Precursors

Many other researchers all over the world have coined their own names for the precursor particles. The name either relates to a unique quality discovered in them because of an action being observed or to where they were found in a certain body in great abundance. For instance, in the 1930s embryologist and biochemist Joseph Needham, Ph.D., observed how these particulates help with cellular individuation during the gestation of frog embryos. Among other things, he was searching for a source of energy inducing cell development. Because of this induction capacity, he called the particles *evocators*.[18]

Renowned English pathologist J. George Adami, M.D., who wrote a foundational handbook on pathology in 1908, developed the concept of a *biophore*, and deemed it the "ultimate molecule of living matter." He believed this was where heredity came from.

In the later nineteenth century, German physician August Weisman, M.D., referred to the precursors as *ancestral plasmas* being passed from generation to generation. He witnessed two forms, one inside the cell and one outside the cell, which he respectively named the *id* and the *idant.*[19]

Scottish Australian pharmacologist and chemist Thorburn Brailsford Robertson, Ph.D., D.Sc., who is best remembered for manufacturing the first insulin for treatment of diabetes in the 1920s wrote in *Biochemical Journal* in 1921 that there is a factor in blood, an *x-substance,* that stimulates the reproduction of cells, including bacteria and yeast. He was referring to the pleomorphism of the precursory particles.[20]

Most recently, in 1991, a Finnish scientist at the University of Kuopio, discovered what he called *nano-bacteria,* showing how they "grow both inside and outside of mammalian cells and show a diameter of 0.2 to 0.3 mm. . . . exhibit a remarkable thermostability . . . produce biogenic apatite, a major constituent of our bones."[21]

There were many others, but perhaps most important was dentist Royal Lee, D.D.S., a visionary engineer and patent holder who has come to be known as one of the fathers of holistic nutrition. Lee understood that the most important factor when it came to disease, repair, and health of the body is nutrition. He was able to connect the dots between nutrient deficiencies and disease progression, starting with defining what tooth decay really was. He saw that though a person may not have outward signs of a deficiency, if that individual is walking around with minimal stores of a vitamin, the deficiency can be causing deterioration of their tissues in subtle ways. He also recognized that this, in turn, significantly affected the pleomorphic activity of the precursors.

Lee observed the research of Edward Rosenow at the Mayo Foundation and was able to determine that the reason behind the pleomorphing of the bacteria was a change in the nutritional content of their growth mediums. Rosenow was culturing his bacteria in a variety of different broths.[22]

Rosenow proved, without a doubt, that bacteria undergo a complete transformation from one type to another—complete in terms of structure, behavior, and specific identifying tendencies. According to an article published in 1955, "He demonstrated transmutations within germs of the pneumonia group."[23] He would take various microbes from different body parts of different animals and humans and put them all in the same type of medium. An example of this was when he took streptococcus and watched it transform into staphylococcus, once placed into a new Petri dish environment, and then back to streptococcus, once returned to original environment. After a while, no scientist could tell them apart. He concluded there was no difference between these two germs.

Rosenow believed, at that time, that his findings would have severe consequences in bacteriology, epidemiology, and medicine because it pointed to the possibility that our bodies created the disease. He wrote that infections should not be used as places of focus for treatment but rather for an understanding of something deficient in the body as a whole.

Rosenow replicated this research thousands of times and it was also replicated and verified by other scientists all over the world.

Lee subsequently studied the precursors himself and named them *protomorphogens*, which, loosely translated, means the "primitive material from which an organ is created." His understanding of the protomorphogens was at the same level as many other researchers and microscopists of the time. And Lee determined, as they did, that all biological growth is controlled and maintained by these precursors. Furthermore, he was able to connect the production of bacteria—the middle stage of the pleomorphic cycle—to a lack of particular nutrients, dependent on body symptoms and signs.

A modern scientist can easily disregard many of the experiments of antiquity, yet pleomorphism happens not only to simple microorganisms, but also to many multicellular organisms around them. That cannot be as easily disregarded. Animals like frogs, butterflies, and even humans go through various stages of change, pleomorphism, some more extreme than others in their growth. While humans change in size and reproductive capabilities outside of the womb, frogs change in such extreme ways, having tails and living in water to developing limbs and living on land, losing the ability to survive underwater and adjusting to living on land.

There are actual recent studies in support of pleomorphism, and these scientists went to considerable lengths to demonstrate the purity of their experiments. Late-twentieth-century studies show the morphology change in *Thiobacillus* in response to the environment. Other papers from as recently as a couple decades ago show complex life cycles and universal *endoparasitism* with bacteria passing through these various stages in the cycle.[24]

Stuart Grace writes: "The debate today should not be over whether pleomorphism exists. Our efforts should focus on the attempt to understand the biological mechanisms, evolutionary origins, and practical, clinical applications of these remarkable capabilities."[25]

In her book, *Cell Wall Deficient Forms: Stealth Pathogens*, which was originally published in 1974, immunologist Lida H. Mattman, Ph.D., describes her research on bacterial variability, documenting changes in morphology and metabolism. She states, with "carefully prepared pure cultures, [I] found that bacteria pass through stages with markedly different morphology."[26] The entire book is about forms of bacteria that lack a cell wall. In it, she mentions the work of many other scientists whose similar discoveries were overlooked or ridiculed despite them having made stringent and complex preparations prior to observation.

More recently physician Maria Bleker, M.D., who upon attending university in the 1950s, heard the news about a scientist, Gunther Enderlein at the time, discovering the endobionts present in all humans. Bearing witness to his work and seeing firsthand the blatant disregard of his "observation-based determination of developmental processes in microbes," led Bleker to do her own research, as many others did and still do and realize that "Enderlein's teachings are not mere 'theory' but rather pure natural knowledge."[27]

It is also worth noting, for conversation purposes, in the scientific community, there lies a problem of communication about pleomorphism since the term now means different things. Some groups believe the word to mean a shedding of their cell walls, while others use it to mean shedding of antigenic markers. How I use it and how it is used here, is how Enderlein and his associates used it, that the precursors give rise successively to more complex forms, bacteria or fungus within the body.

Figure 5.3 is my simplistic visual interpretation of the cycle. Remember within each group there can be thousands if not millions of various forms. This is a generalized expression of possible forms a precursor takes.

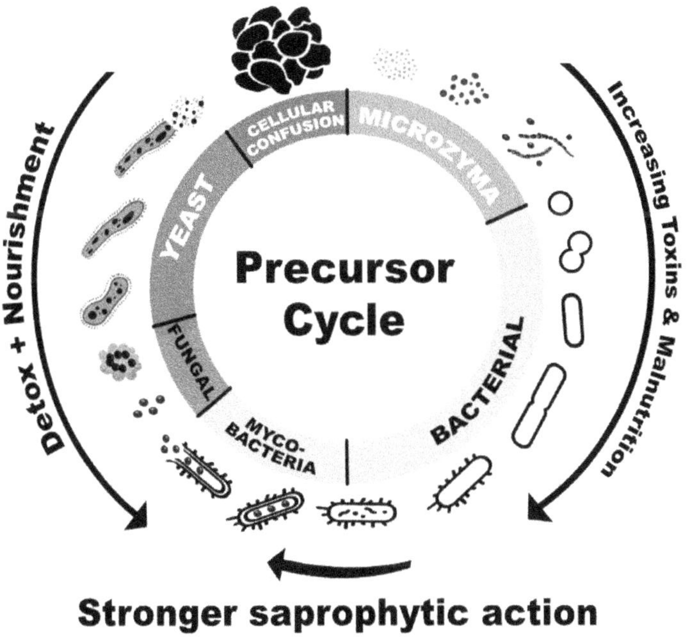

Figure 5.3 The pleomorphic cycle that precursors go through.

Remember, "germs" are just precursors that have evolved into bacteria to do necessary cleanup work in their environment. The precursors transform into the bacteria necessary to clean the specific tissue to which they are exposed. Understanding this, it is easy to realize that if you were to put bacteria in one Petri dish, have the organisms multiply in the culture, and then move the bacteria to another Petri dish containing another type of tissue sample or culture medium, you would see the bacteria change shape.

That was what I was seeing occur when I was doing my graduate studies in microbiology. And this is essentially what is happening in our bodies every day as we are exposed to food, air, water, and many other types of stressors. We owe the precursors a debt of gratitude for their support.

SIX

THE IMPORTANCE OF THE ENVIRONMENT TO OUR TERRAIN

"The Earth is not the environment, something outside of us that we need to care for. The Earth is us. Taking care of the Earth, we take care of ourselves."

THICH NHAT HANH

Diseases are formed through no fault of the bacteria and fungi in our bodies. Energy, sonic resonance, environmental conditions, astronomical events like solar flares, and other factors may adversely affect our terrain. In this chapter, we will look at how our world has become increasingly polluted and harmful to us in the past hundred years. In particular, as negligence and greed took control of the progression of medicine, simple health-care fixes such as effective sanitation and natural treatments were dismissed though they were nontoxic and tended to cost less than drugs prescribed for common chronic ailments, including arthritis, hypertension, and type 2 diabetes.

Today, industries looking to profit off of newly defined diseases routinely add more toxins to our internal terrain when they provide us with their expensive "cures," drumming up, and then banking on, our societal fear of contagion. Based upon the deception that is the germ theory, vaccines are seen as a panacea. They have proliferated, becoming the only treatment allowed, and are required to attend schools and do certain jobs. Because industrial plants spew pollution into our air, water, and soil, illness flourishes. Our world is now a web of profits and lies.

The moment scientists discovered that microbes are dependent on their environment to adaptively change their forms, the important role that the environment plays in affecting the well-being of living organisms, including human beings, became evident. Three researchers led the research: Royal Rife, Günther Enderlein, and Gaston Naessens. They discovered the various forms microbes take using specific types of microscopes that they themselves invented for this purpose. These microscopes can show, without a doubt, how precursors in several different types of media, are able to change form and create new dimensions of their existence.

Stages of the Pleomorphic Cycle

If you were merely to peer into a darkfield microscope, which essentially is a light microscope with a darkfield oil condenser that is easily accessible to any layperson, you would be able to see the forms of the precursors developing over time as the cells within your sample slowly died. I've observed this phenomenon myself many, many times.

Many scientists have tediously and exhaustively gone through the process of observing the multitude of forms that arise from changing the environment of precursors. Observers have included Antoine Béchamp, Günther Enderlein, Ernst Almquist, Royal Rife, and Gaston Naessens. Almquist, together with Robert Koch, also made observations about assorted forms of microorganisms in their typhoid fever patients. Although Koch then made attempts to simplify his explanation for what he was witnessing when he saw the forms, Almquist came to the conclusion: "Nobody can pretend to know the complete life cycle and all the varieties of even a single bacterial species."[1] He went on to discover spontaneous forms arising in people suffering from symptoms associated with various other diseases.

The Effect of an Unhealthy Environment on Pleomorphism

Some scientists recognize the phenomenon of pleomorphism and still subscribe to germ theory. Dr. Enderlein was one such researcher. He believed that after a certain point of development, precursors in their bacterial form that are transforming into the form of a fungus are contributing to the pathogenicity of the body, creating secondary and even tertiary ailments. Enderlein believed to have witnessed the eventual breakdown of healthy tissue by the destructive forces of highly pathogenic fungi in the pleomorphic cycle. But I believe he failed to interpret what he was seeing correctly because his research was done on blood in a laboratory and he never interacted with patients directly, along with mistaking signs of inflammation like endotoxins/ exotoxins as stimulators for better regulation rather than deterioration. His observations were steeped in the observance of blood in an entirely clinical setting and not contingent on the context of healthy dietary conditions, such as a hygienic home, proper nutrition, and fresh water.

Though Enderlein may have believed in the pleomorphic cycle that the *protits* (precursors) in his laboratory engaged in, he never incorporated the influence of nature itself on the blood he was studying in the lab. He simply did not understand the importance of the dynamic between the protits and the external milieu in which they existed. Nor did he recognize the mutualism of homeostasis for which the precursors and the human body depend on each other.

By *mutualism*, I mean the way our internal microbiomes help to clean and maintain our bodies all the while we maintain the integrity of our internal environments with a healthy diet and lifestyle.

In a way, Antoine Béchamp did not fully comprehend that either, being that he was more focused on identifying the *microzymas* within living and dead matter than on studying their exact influence on the human body when exposed to various circumstances and outer stimuli.

The problem with not understanding the factors that might damage the body, such as toxicity and malnutrition, is that one cannot properly study living matter if one doesn't have the capacity to discern differences between healthy tissue samples and unhealthy ones. Even today, with our advanced equipment, scientists have trouble identifying unhealthy tissue through the lenses of a microscope. Minute changes occur long before damage becomes severe. It is within the comparison of knowing optimally healthy versus barely correctly functioning that much has been missed.

Studies on the virulence of end-stage forms of the pleomorphic cycle whose results are based solely on lab assessments may be missing out on important data. Let's remember, movement through the cycle for the precursors happens as a result of their placement in hostile terrain, as E.C. Rosenow of the Mayo Clinic proved.

Louis Pasteur unknowingly proved that same point by running many experiments in which he introduced strains of microbes to the bodies of animals and measured the presence of the microbes afterward to see if the strains he was using were pathogenic—viewing them in a Petri dish through a microscope. In this scenario, the idea was that a "strong" strain would overwhelm a "weak" strain. But because the microbes were undergoing pleomorphism, his results apparently confused him. He saw evidence he interpreted as diminished pathogenicity, which was really evidence of the precursors adapting to their new environment. This outcome occurred because pleomorphism was happening after each introduction of the microbes to a new animal in the lab. The body was reacting with its customary physiological measures to the unnatural presence of foreign material in order to reestablish its homeostasis.

Enderlein's research captured evidence of this phenomenon as well. He formulated *isopathic remedies*, which work on the premise that precursors adapt to the terrain. When an active form of a precursor in a high-valance form, like a bacterium, is introduced into the body, the bacterium isopathically regresses to a lower valence, inactive form in the presence of passive forms of the same type.

As the precursors move forward in the cycle of transformation that we call *pleomorphic reorganization* and become higher-valence forms so that they may complete their cleanup tasks, they become less "scrupulous" and will begin to break down tissue that has even the slightest indication of corruption in it. This is what we have interpreted as *pathogenicity.* How can this be argued when we know that, in all of nature, parasites and predators alike consume what is weakest or most broken down, not the other way around?

Ill Health, Deficiency, and the Parasitic Tendency

Can we truly measure the level of health inside the body, scientifically? My view is no. You would have to take an inventory of every single cell in the body—trillions of them—and be able to determine down to the level of replication that a cell is functioning at close to 100 percent capacity. Science cannot do that. Yet naturopaths, hygienists, chiropractors, homeopaths, doctors, and healers of old, despite not knowing the specificity of people's cell on a microscopic level, managed to know by observation and the use of the scientific method how to assess the general state of a person's health on a level we cannot in our day. Modern-day conventional tools for measuring how well or poorly different systems of the body are functioning are limited in terms of studying the behavior of the microorganisms that live within us.

To believe even for one second that we hold within us a multitude of organisms lying in wait to destroy their own niche in our bodies, or render it useless, is to deny our recognition of the intelligence that created the human body.

Enderlein created his chart of the pleomorphic cycle, or *bacterial cyclogeny*, as he referred to it, without taking the terrain of the body into account as a pertinent influence to its framework. That is the failure of understanding that most people in the germ theory camp have, and, there are some in the terrain camp, like Enderlein, that still blame the saprophytes for creating our symptoms at one point or another.

It is most important to understand that the precursors, no matter their level of strength or where they are in their pleomorphic cycle are there to facilitate our bodies in restoring or maintaining homeostasis, not to detract from it or add to an imbalance.

Another argument that some people against the complete use of the terrain model are having is about the reason we see an increased bacterial load at the end stage of many diseases. Some people view the increased symptoms, such as weakness of the sick person and an excessive production of microorganisms like bacteria, to be detrimental. But in my view, and in the views of many other followers of the terrain model, these observers are misguidedly interpreting the weakness as making the body a more welcoming host for microorganisms. They think weakness leaves the door open for "opportunistic" and "aggressive" microbes. This doesn't jive with my understanding of the symbiotic relationship between our terrain and the precursors in and around it.

Is the notion of *opportunistic microorganisms* not germ theory again? Have those who propose this idea delicately reincorporated germ theory into their answer to the question of why we see so many bacteria when we're feeling sick? In my opinion, they have because they do not understand the existence of the precursors and the magnitude of malnutrition in the body of that *afflicted* person.

In fact, the precursors are ubiquitous, as proven by the observations of Antoine Béchamp and Wilhelm Reich—respectively of microzymas and bions. They both calculated that ten or more precursors exist for every cell in the body.

Consider the idea that if even just half of those precursors converted into simple bacteria, the body, in the conventional sense, would be overrun with severe infection. What we are seeing in an end-stage disease, therefore, is the picture of the precursors working at their full capacity, with the body's resources almost exhausted (most likely due to a lack of proper nutrition and support, and perhaps due to chemical exposure to medications that further interfere with the whole process of detoxification and repair). The pendulum of homeostasis will always want to swing back to health, and it is only outside interference that inhibits or alters that process.

On the other hand, what's occurring in the presence of parasites—protozoa and helminths (worms)—may be a slightly different story. (There is a contention that these type of multicellular organisms, like other precursors, can be grown inside of us, depending on the toxicity of the terrain. Though this can be true, it may also be true that one can be host to these parasites when conditions are met in the body to ensure the necessity of their existence there.)

The way modern science explains how we become hosts to parasites is not entirely accurate. For instance, science says that parasites take and never give. This is wrong. In actuality, the presence of parasites can be beneficial to us even as they serve their own interests. For a parasite to want to take advantage of your body, you would have to be malnourished due to the type of loss of resources that occurs when a toxic load has not been fully excreted. The body can become nutritionally deficient when it's trying to repair damage from exposure to toxins. If you are healthy, then you simply won't be as attractive to parasites.

Leeches are great examples of parasites that provide benefits to their hosts. All the while they are drinking their host's blood, they are removing dead tissue and improving blood flow for the host. For this reason, leeches are utilized in the reattachment of severed digits and ears.[2]

In nature, predators always seek weakness, which ultimately serves the surviving members of a defending species. We know, for instance, that in the case of a mosquito or tick, you have to be deficient in B vitamins to attract the insects to bite you.[3] In addition, the terrain has to be able to host other types of parasites, giving them an appropriate setting in which to thrive and reproduce.

Not all people who consume meat that has tapeworm eggs in it become infected with tapeworms. Therefore we can conclude that even when we are exposed to a parasite, if we are in good standing nutrition-wise, have limited to no toxic metals in our bodies, and have developed a good balance of life within us, parasites will be of no consequence to us. Interestingly, certain intestinal worms consume vast quantities of certain heavy metals, leaving the surrounding tissue devoid of those materials. In a study done looking at intestinal parasites, namely various helminths (multicellular worms) in urban rats, a "higher concentration of heavy metals were revealed in the helminths than in the host tissues . . . more than ten-fold higher,"[4] clearly showing how much toxins these city rats are exposed to.

So, are these parasites really "parasitic" or are they working symbiotically with the host environment?

As you have read, precursors are all around us and within us, possibly to the extent of ten for every cell. From the toxins in our bodies to the decaying material in a forest, our world requires their existence and abilities to exist. As they progress in their cycle to become the consumers of garbage (*saprophytes*), our bodies supply them with necessary help, be it in the form of white blood cells or diversion of enzymes, to name a couple of physiological examples. Yet, even some people that subscribe to the terrain paradigm still hold bacteria, fungi, and even viruses culpable for contributing to and exacerbating disease conditions, potentially even complicating our disease states. This exacerbation or complication is assumed to be caused by an increase in virulence, the production of either endotoxins or exotoxins, and an elevated presence of microbes.

But I ask, if it is a bacterium's job to clean up a mess in our body, why would it add to the mess it is trying to eliminate? From an adaptation standpoint, what would be the point of an organism overrunning a delicate habitat?

In their book, *What Really Makes Us Ill?* citizen scientists Dawn Lester and David Parker write:

> *It is the contention of some people, particularly in the "alternative health" community, that bacteria only become pathogenic under certain conditions; that they only play a secondary role in disease. This view claims that bacteria are not the original cause of disease, but that they proliferate as the direct result of disease. It is further claimed that it is the proliferation of the bacteria that directly contributes to the worsening of the diseases due to the "toxins" released by these "bad" bacteria. The idea that "bacterial toxins" are the causes of many illnesses is fundamentally flawed; the main reason is due to the normal presence in the body of many trillions of bacteria. If only a tiny percentage of the trillions of bacteria in the body produced "toxins," people would always be ill, from the moment of birth and throughout their entire lives. If any of these toxins were truly "deadly," it raises the question of how life could ever have begun, considering that bacteria are one of the earliest "life forms."*[5]

Remember, the precursors are there, changing and shifting to respond to the internal environment and help maintain its well-being. Their form adapts to respond to stressors. If they deem it necessary, more of them will cycle into the type of organisms necessary to handle the responsibility of cleaning up. This does not mean they are adding to the degeneracy of the body; rather, they are trying to expedite a cleansing process.

Pleomorphism and the Terrain Model Go Hand in Hand

Let's get one thing clear: Just because someone believes in pleomorphism doesn't necessarily mean they believe in the terrain model. There are several "pleomorphists" who believe in the germ theory, and there are several "monomorphists" who believe in the terrain model, truly only getting part of the picture. The idea is to understand that pleomorphism and the terrain model are dependent on one another, which means that you cannot believe in the terrain in its whole essence without completely understanding pleomorphism, and you can't understand pleomorphism in its whole essence without understanding the terrain model. Many studies have proved the fact that changing the environment alters the appearance of the bacteria and fungi living in it. Furthermore, as early as 1913, research showed that there are *progressive* stages of transmutation.[6]

Energy and Resonance, and Their Influence on Human Beings

Without detouring into the topic of quantum physics, let's do our best to understand our physical structure on the microscopic level. At this level, we are essentially all made up of atoms, which, in turn, are composed of neutrons, protons, and electrons. If you do any reading in science, then you know that electrons are negatively charged particles that spin around the core or *nucleus* of an atom (made up of protons and neutrons) forming a *shell* that looks like a cloud because of the speed at which the electrons move.

Electrons can travel. They can stay close to their nucleus, inside the body, or with sufficient energy to break their nuclear bond, they can move almost infinitely far from the physical body. In doing so, these electrons expand to great distances, interacting with electrons belonging to atoms in other people and objects. Therefore each of us is constantly interacting with the atoms of our environment, objects, and people, sometimes over vast distances.

Each physical object in existence that contains atoms has a plume of electrons swimming in a cloud about it. In certain fields of study, it's believed that the electron cloud is the same thing as what spiritualists term the *aura*. The electrons in this energy field are moving at a certain pace: sometimes fast, sometimes slow, based on the activity of the main object, which in the case of this discussion is the human body. At different speeds, electrons generate different frequencies of energy.

At times, such as when our electrons have a chance to interact with electrons from another source, they have a tendency to be influenced by them, meaning they will speed up or slow their spinning action depending on what the other electrons are doing, especially if both sets of electrons are similar in their actions.

This influence changes the electron action and reverberates the action throughout the atom. This ripple effect continues with a million more atoms and will show up eventually on a bigger scale, first within molecules, then bigger particles, and then eventually cells in the body.

This is an oversimplified explanation, showing a possibility for why people are influenced, even at a distance, by people around them. Imagine the scenario of someone yawning. A behavior whose purpose is still undefined by science, when one person yawns other people tend to imitate the behavior. Animals do this too.

Another helpful example of electron communication is the phenomenon of tuning forks vibrating together. When a tuning fork is set at a certain frequency, it vibrates when struck, making a tonal sound. Let's say a 440-Hz tuning fork is struck and creates the sound of the A note above middle C. If there is a nearby tuning fork that resonates at 493 Hz (a middle B), there is little to no impact on that particular fork because it doesn't share the same frequency. The waves of the air and the electrons around the tuning fork are not being stimulated to move at the 440 Hz frequency.

But if there are any tuning forks in the vicinity of the original 440-Hz tuning fork that correspond to the same Hz, they will start to ring, even without having a physical exchange. When two objects vibrate at the same frequency, we say they are "on the same wavelength."

Of course, vibrations are occurring beyond the spectrum of sound audible to us. Other creatures, like bats and whales, can perceive tones that are either higher or lower than the average human ear can perceive. Resonance helps us realize how nonphysical communication of energy occurs even when we cannot consciously see, hear, or are aware of an electron changing its orientation.

For me, the science of vibrations explains our misunderstanding of contagion. And why some people exhibit the same symptoms after interacting with another person who is "sick." Each of their bodies is, in a way, resonating at the same wavelength. This communication of electrons, through resonance, frequency, and so on, signals to the other person's body to commence with the same detoxification symptoms.

This phenomenon can be measured in the similar patterning of people's bodies, whether it is people who live in the same house, in the same town, or of the same gender, or even the same ethnicity. An example is menstruation. When women gather together regularly, a form of communication happens in their bodies so they get their periods simultaneously. Though mistakenly considered pheromones, it is still uncertain by modern science as to what exactly is being communicated between ovulating women.

As olfactory researcher Richard L. Doty, Ph.D., Director of the University of Pennsylvania's Smell and Taste Center, states: "Attempts to identify mammalian pheromones have been generally unsuccessful, regardless as to whether such agents are viewed as releaser pheromones, priming pheromones, modulating pheromones, or any other type of putative pheromone."[7]

Recall the yawning example. We exhibit the same type of reaction in our own bodies when we see a person yawn, but *only if* we are already tired or hungry or mineral deficient. You could be watching a person yawn on television or talking to them on the phone, sitting next to them, or saying hello on the street. They yawn and you yawn.

There are also theories that DNA is resonant and contains a frequency, or possibly is *itself* a frequency. In 2011, *International Journal of Radiation Biology* published the report of a study in which chromosomes are referred to as *fractal antennae*.[8] Being that we leave our DNA everywhere—in the air and on whatever we touch or interact with—its influence potentially creates changes in other people's bodies. The frequency of our DNA may be one of the media for communication that our bodies use. Do you remember Gunther Enderlein? He theorized, by witnessing it happening in his microscope, that the same precursors he saw transforming into their various forms (*endobionts*, he called them) were actually the DNA in each cell. This finding correlates with his observations about endobiont inheritance and immortality.

All these things are examples of ways the body engages in resonant communication. In 2002, James Gimzewski and Andrew Pelling, using an atomic force microscope, were able to amplify and pick up the sounds from cells, inventing the science of *sonocytology* in the process. The sound of an individual cell's metabolism resembles squealing. Apparently, the cells in our bodies "sing" to one another, engaging in a grand communication on a level we have yet to understand.[9]

When the cells and the tissue alike are healthy and happy, they produce a harmonious resonance that is amplified by each cell that is working cooperatively. When they are sickly or working against each other, the "singing" becomes more discordant.

In addition to the effects of energetic frequencies on the human body, the body is affected by astronomical events, like solar wind, sunspots, and the movements of the sun, moon, and various other planetary bodies. If this seems farfetched, please remember that inside the body there exists a whole figurative universe, teeming with organisms and processes, many yet to be discovered and most that have been discovered yet to be fully explained. Just as many cultures have learned how to yield certain crops in great quantity by planting seedlings during a full moon, we too, due to the presence of precursors inside us, can be affected by atmospheric and astronomical changes.

Take the work of H. Bortels, who was the director of bacteriology at Berlin University, in the 1930s. He reported discovering a "constant factor in his test tubes and cultures of bacilli: the shift from high to low pressure and from a warm to a cold front in the atmosphere altered the behavior of the microbes to a considerable extent."[10] Yet when he protected one group from the sunlight in a lead/iron box, the activity of being affected by atmospheric and weather changes, ceased to be.

Another example of mysterious influences is when biologist Frank A. Brown, Ph.D., a professor at Northwestern University, studied colloids suspended in water, "in a uniform environment . . . mysteriously informed of changes in certain external factors."[11] This begs the question as to where the information could possibly derive from, could it be those ubiquitous, barely seen precursors?

Twentieth-century Russian-Polish biophysicist Alexander Tchijewsky of Moscow University noted how there was something in the air to cure ailments. In 1926, he purchased a very sickly chimpanzee, in the last stages of tuberculosis, close to death, but within four months turned the health of the animal completely around, which then lived on for many more years. Tchijewsky believed that in teaching the chimpanzee deep breathing, he was able to infuse the animals lungs maximally with life-giving particles, which he regarded as "negative ions" in the air. Professor Tchijewsky was a pioneer in the study of charged particles in the air. He also believed these particles to be influenced by an eleven-year solar cycle that he correlated with a 72 percent accuracy to epidemics, wars, and revolutions.[12]

The same eleven-year sunspot cycle sparked the attention of another scientist, Maki Takata, M.D., a professor at

Toho university in Tokyo, Japan, who, in 1928, created a method to test for a phenomenon in the bloodstream now known as the *Takata reaction*. With many doctors worldwide using his test to analyze women's ovarian cycles, he discovered that a protein in the blood of both men and women responds to fluctuations in solar activity: solar flares, storms, sunrise, sunset, and the eleven-year sunspot cycle.[13]

Our society has known that temperature and air quality affect our health for hundreds of years, as was pointed out two hundred years ago by American physician James Clark, M.D., when he wrote: "The influence of climate over disease has been long established as a matter of fact, and physicians have, from a very early period, considered change of climate and change of air as remedial agents of great efficacy. . . . It may suffice to mention here, in reference to this fact, intermittent fevers, asthma, catarrhal affections, whooping cough . . . These diseases are often benefited, and not infrequently cured, by simple change of situation, after having long resisted medical treatment."[14]

The terrain model appreciates and embraces this idea of communication and interaction. When the person's body is similar in health and structure to another person's body and either person is in the midst or at the beginning of detoxification—which is conventionally known as *sickness*—it will signal to one another. This can happen on the small scale of two individuals or on the grand scale of an entire country. Whether communication occurs via a visual cue, a chemical excretion, an electron cloud, or even the sharing of water or sun particles, there is a signal.

When you die and your body disintegrates, only dust is left over, whether you are buried and decay or you are cremated. This dust goes back into the soil. Even as corpses, we have communicating precursors. My "guys" are going to talk to your "guys."

Remember, the electron shell of an atom is like a plume that encircles the atom; this energy, which exudes from every single atom in every molecule in our bodies, comingles with the electron clouds of the atoms in molecules of every other thing it touches.

Like electrons in their atomic clouds, precursors are floating around our cells. Precursors are indestructible beings that cannot die. They are part of our bodies. They coexist with us. They are something that cannot be measured for which conventional science has to date attributed no value.

When Béchamp performed an experiment of removing or flushing the precursors (aka microzymas) from a cell, the cell immediately died. He did this experimentally to a piece of meat, and it decayed more rapidly than normal. He also put a dead cat in a glass case, an enclosed environment, where neither flies nor airborne contaminants could touch it and the corpse took seven years to decompose. All that was left from this experiment was white dust.

Everyone naturally inquired, "How did the cat's body break down?" The answer is that the breakdown was initiated from within the animal. Those particles, the precursors, were breaking everything down for seven years.

Then, when they were done, they reverted from their bacterial form back to their crystalline dust state.

From ashes to ashes, dust to dust.

SEVEN

HOW DO VIRUSES FIT THE TERRAIN MODEL?

"In the sciences, people quickly come to regard as their own personal property that which they have learned and had passed on to them at the universities and academies. If however, someone else now comes along with new ideas that contradict the Credo (that has been recited for years and passed on in turn to others) and in fact even threaten to overturn it, then all passions are raised against this threat and no method is left untried to suppress it."

JOHANN WOLFGANG VON GOETHE

Russian bacteria hunter Dimitri Iwanowski, who gathered fluid from diseased tobacco plants in 1892, is said to have achieved the first isolation of a virus. He passed his liquid through a filter fine enough to retain bacteria, yet to Iwanowski's surprise, the bacteria-free filtrate nonetheless made healthy plants sick. But what made the plants sick? He decided it was a form of micro-organism smaller than bacteria.

In reviewing Iwanowski's research, it doesn't seem as if he considered the possibility that poisonous excretions or disrupted energy in the proteins of the diseased cells had made the other plants sick, which is how a terrain doctor such as me would explain the same phenomenon.

Since Iwanowski's discovery of nonfilterable particles, which supposedly were "organisms," later named *viruses*, researchers in different fields have attributed diseases to super tiny particles if they could not find bacteria, fungi, or parasitic organisms to blame. In fact, there were particles present in the liquid, but he misidentified them as contagious, half-living parasites.

To this day, conventional science has settled the science through consensus that viruses exist, yet to many microbiologists around the world, including virologists, there are quite a number of unanswered questions as to whether or not they exist at all, since they are only seen through induced or contrived means in laboratories and have never actually been singled out in any real, natural environment.

Furthermore, although they have been studied at length by researchers, how they function inside the bodies of their "hosts" (if we agree they are parasitic) is still a mystery since the only way to observe them is through the lens of an electron microscope. There are problems with this method of research. Virus hunters conveniently ignore a pivotal principle of scientific methodology in the design of their experiments: Ideally, there should be complete purification of viral material from a source prior to testing or identification. They have not accomplished it.[1]

How an Electron Microscope Works

To study a virus, one must view it through the lens of an electron microscope—it is *that* small. Unfortunately, the method of preparation of materials to be viewed in this manner damages the samples. The sample that is assumed to have a virus, be it saliva or some other excretion, is not purified but rather added and grown in a toxic medium, something, is removed, again an assumed organism, stains and toxic dehydrating substances are further added, and then it is suspended in a resin to suspend and hold the sample. Thus, an electron microscope can only give us a snapshot of what is happening *after* preparation has occurred.

Unfortunately, the medium that is used in preparation of samples is toxic to living tissue. Therefore, a researcher would never be able to discern, for example, whether a protein they are looking at on a slide was captured as it was entering a cell or as it was leaving it. If the researcher saw a protein in the sample they would have to guess at the reason for its presence.

Here is a second troubling issue related to the same technology. A scanning electron microscope (SEM) is a kind of electron microscope that works by sending an accelerated beam of electrons toward a specimen that was prepared by a technician. This beam is created by 100,000 volts of electricity. The images the technician sees on a view screen are made by the electrons reaction to various substances. But it is impossible to ascertain whether the electrons bombarded reflect, penetrate, or get absorbed by the material without staining.

Just like a sample assumed to contain a virus, suspended in a toxic chemical medium are not alive, the specimens in this type of analysis are not alive either. No living organism would be able to survive once it was exposed to the preparation materials prior to being viewed in a microscope or to receiving volts of electricity during the scanning. Furthermore, due to both these processes, the state of the nonliving material is also likely to be degraded and so is not an accurate representation of any organism in its living state.

Many specimens prepared for the electron microscope undergo a sequence of chemical exposures in order to stabilize them. The first is a bath in glutaraldehyde and/or formaldehyde. This starts the fixation process. The tissue or fluid being studied typically stays immersed in this chemical for one to three hours.

Second, a contrasting agent is added. Usually osmium tetroxide, which is so poisonous it would blind us if it got in our eyes. This chemical enables different features to be seen on the screen.

The third step, dehydration, is done to ensure the specimen is completely devoid of water molecules. Acetone or other drying chemicals are used along with carbon dioxide flushing, to enhance the drying agents.

The next step is to embed the tissue sample, or what's left of it after the chemical baths, into a liquid resin that is heated at 320 degrees Fahrenheit for either a couple of hours or a day to harden it. Then it is sectioned, which is slicing it in a specific way.

Yet another chemical is added before examination, either uranyl acetate or lead citrate—and occasionally both. A slice of the fixed specimen is then placed into the electron microscope where it is exposed to massive amounts of electrons.[2]

The toxic soup that samples of tissue are prepared with, which I've just described, is considered a standard for looking at anything too tiny to be seen through the lenses of a regular optical microscope. There are other methods used to prepare tissue samples, too, like certain freeze-drying techniques, and these involve the immersion of the specimen in a chemical, either ethanol, tertiary butanol, phosphate-buffered saline, formalin, liquid carbon dioxide, or liquid platinum. Afterward, the sample is subjected to intense pressure and heat.[3]

Microscopes Don't Prove the Existence of Viruses

Not a single virus is ever viewed in a live state, only in the special way the electron microscopist uses. Almost all the images the public sees of a virus are computer-generated fabrications that assume what the virus is doing to a cell based on interpretations of snapshots from microscopes.

This is the equivalent of taking a snapshot of a person running from a store. Is the individual running away from the store because he stole something or running out of the store to chase after a criminal? Is he running away from somebody chasing him? Is he just going for a jog because he likes to run? We cannot tell from a glance. The interpretation depends on the narrative an observer goes by. It is fictional.

The level of conjecture in the field of virology has reached the point that almost all information given would be deemed less than circumstantial if presented to a judge in a court case. That's not a lot to go on, yet medicine still expends billions of dollars in researching, fighting, and inoculating against something they know less than 1 percent about.

In the late 1980s, Peter Duesberg, Ph.D., a professor of molecular and cell biology at the University of California, realized that many viruses which were suspected of causing diseases were not being found in many patients. Thousands of AIDS patients, for instance, never had HIV in their bodies.[4] His interpretation of what causes AIDS symptoms is wildly different from the mainstream explanation other doctors accept. Duesberg believes that symptoms of AIDS are chemically induced by drugs people consume, whether illicit or prescribed.

Another idea that has been presented as an explanation for the presence of viruses in micrographs is that they are, in fact, *exosomes*, small, single-membrane, secreted organelles anywhere from 30 and 200 nanometers (a billionth of a meter) in diameter which have the same topology as cells and are enriched in proteins, lipids, nucleic acids, and glycoconjugates.[5] These excretions of a dying cell may be what electron microscopes are viewing. This seems plausible to me since the cells would have died while being prepared for viewing, though this is not proof of their existence in nature or in natural circumstances within the body.

Or perhaps exosomes are actually precursors, rather than the innards of cells! This is a possibility if one looks at the extensive work of Dr. Gunther Enderlein. His analysis of the various pleomorphic forms that occur prior to precursors (*protits*, in his vernacular) transforming into bacteria show that these forms all look like parts of a cell. Enderlein came to the realization that precursors are the foundation of cellular manufacturing by witnessing the formations of what seemed to be stem cell-like cells from the various forms of the precursors in many stages coming together as a community, almost like a small city.

Another scientist, biologist Stephen Lanka, Ph.D., has described what is mistaken as a virus as particles that arose from physical or chemical damage to the cell, basically a byproduct of cellular death. He has asserted that there has never been a "real and complete virus . . . anywhere" in scientific literature.[6]

What Is a Virus, Really

Let me briefly explain the nature of viruses(since they have yet to be proven to cause any negative effect on biological organisms), coming from the perspective of a terrain doctor: Just like bacteria and fungi, you cannot catch them. Dead and dying cells possibly make these particles in the process of dying, excreting them in part to get rid of poisons.

Remember this has still not been proven in living tissue. However, if the body is filled with "garbage," be it dead tissue, some kind of toxin, the byproducts of metabolized hormones, or anything else that the body doesn't want that has not been successfully flushed out through the normal channels of excretion, then the cells will create another method to get rid of them. When they reach sufficient quantities, the body responds with cold- or flu-like symptoms. Cellular excretion gets ramped up so much that the whole body responds.

What is termed *virus production* by mainstream science might just be a multifaceted reaction to an overwhelming influx of toxicity in the body.

A simple analogy to help us understand this phenomenon is what happens when someone gets a splinter. Let's say you got a splinter in your finger, and left it in the skin rather than plucking it out. In a few days, the entrance through which the splinter entered your finger will have closed up. Then the body will employ its own special method for expelling the foreign material. It starts by encompassing the material in a bubble of liquid. This bubble, along with the rapid shedding of skin, slowly pushes the splinter out. When the bubble comes to the surface of the skin, either due to friction or just natural shedding of layers of skin, the bubble opens and the foreign object is released.

This liquid is the main component for removing the splinter. It works to buffer the body against the damage. The foreign object is what we consider a *toxin*, something aggressive enough to disturb the body's equilibrium to the point that a reaction becomes necessary.

Likewise, if there is signaling from cells that they have toxic material outside or within them, the same reaction occurs: bubbling or blistering occurs to remove the harmful material before a whole organ shuts down. Therefore, in the view of terrain medicine, what is seen as *viral material* is most likely only a production instigated by whatever toxin is present. Signaling to remove the noxious material has started to harm or degrade the body by the time we can observe this response.

Never forget, the body naturally wants to stay alive. It therefore produces reactions designed to clean up its tissues and return it to homeostasis.

A noxious material could be *exogenous*, meaning "coming from the outside," such as a chemical or a fake ingredient found in processed food; or it could be *endogenous*, meaning "something coming from the inside," such as dead cells or metabolites that were not broken down properly.

In their book *What Really Makes You Ill?*, British citizen scientists Dawn Lester and David Parker point out that the way science is conducted due to believing in germ theory colors our opinion of our body's natural detoxification mechanisms. They write: "The reason that cell death is perceived to be a 'disease process' is because that is what is likely to have been observed during the laboratory experiments. However, there are genuine reasons for cells to die after tissue samples have been subjected to the various preparation procedures used in the laboratory experimentation."[7]

In their book, *The Contagion Myth*, Thomas S. Cowan, M.D., and Sally Fallon Morell, founding president of the Weston A. Price Foundation, say that "these particles [precursors] are an integral part of our detoxification system. They are the true firemen, obviously present in higher amounts in cases of disease, in which a higher burden of poisoning has occurred."[8] Embracing the premise that the precursors are fundamentally the helpers and cleaners of the cells, inside and out, these authors believe that this is what is captured in resin specimens studied via electron microscopes.

Since none of us live in isolation, being that we are a species that lives in families and communities, all of us are constantly exposed to many factors that affect our health. Within a household, a family generally eats in the same way, is exposed to the same air, and so on. The same thing goes for members of small communities. Environmental factors, such as humidity, variations of temperature, and wind affect everyone in a particular area universally. This is not to mention artificial disruptions in an environment, such as the presence of a power grid, cellular repeaters, and crop treatments, like spraying with pesticides, as well as airplane exhaust, that are airborne. The symptoms that arise with these changes and exposures are what medicine has assumed to be "a virus."

Also don't forget how the sun and psychologically impactful changes in our lives can disrupt our regulatory processes and stimulate the precursors that keep the balance of the body to respond. With factors like stress added to that mix, you have the body producing all sorts of hormones quite erratically.

In my opinion, these commonalities are why we see many people detoxing simultaneously or within a slightly offset time frame. Some people are affected by a heat wave or cold spell and some are not. Some are sensitive to electromagnetism and some are not. We all have separate and distinct reactions to different factors, some stronger than others, because, for the most part, our nutrient health level and our abilities to excrete the toxins efficiently and immediately vary.

The detoxification process is not something that the body wants to resort to frequently, given that it utilizes a lot of energy. During the process, many organs, and sometimes the whole bodily system, can be pushed to exhaustion if unsupported—especially in cases of heavy removal of excretory material. That energy drain is why many people feel (and look) sick and tired periodically. Times like these are when they say they "have caught" or are "battling" a virus.

Precursors are the essential communicators of processes happening within and outside every cell. When precursors in a cell instruct the cell to die, the cell expires. As it does, it releases some of its "innards," including nucleic proteins, which is how the need for detoxification is communicated to the body.[9]

Although the factors that produced our synergy with the billions of organisms cohabitating within us cannot be measured or qualified in any way yet that is sufficient to make dogmatic scientists happy, if we could employ a darkfield microscope to view the world, we would see that everything, including everything we can touch and the whole of the air around us, is covered with precursors. Precursors are the progenitors of life, all other organisms that exist on Earth.[10] Immortal and indestructible, they surround every single cell. Inside the body, they look like infinite stars in the sky through a microscope. If you take them away from a cell, as Antoine Béchamp showed through his experiments, then the cell dies.[11]

Precursors in one of their activated forms could be what scientists generally see in their microscopes when they believe they have seen viruses—not attackers, but helpful organisms trying to fix the body.

And if you were wondering, they're not seeing nucleic proteins either, because nucleic proteins are too small to view in a microscope.

Vaccines and the Immune System Fiction

One of the greatest debates we have in our era is whether or not vaccines work. This book is not here to weigh in on that subject. But, on one level, it is intended to help you understand how the science of terrain medicine likely invalidates the need to use vaccines altogether. If viruses do not exist (and again, whether they do or don't, *they are not harmful)*, and if microbes are here to help remove toxins, do we really need vaccines?

As a terrain doctor, it is my belief that the body has mechanisms to protect itself from being damaged by toxins. These include organs of digestion and elimination, like the kidneys, the liver, and the gut, as well as the lungs and the skin. The body works in different ways to isolate toxicity, inflaming respective systems, and thereby triggering them to flush out the toxins that the body so desperately needs to get rid of. This inflammation and detoxification occurs with the assistance of precursors going through their various changes to adapt to the needs of the body, which will be different in any given moment.

Because the precursors and our own detoxification systems have our needs covered, vaccinations are unnecessary. Furthermore, they are potentially damaging. If we take a look at some of the substances that are injected into people's bodies as vaccines, we find plenty of *adjuvant* ingredients in them, substances intended to modulate or increase the body's response to the vaccine. Given the presence of things like aluminum hydroxide, aluminum phosphate, and aluminum potassium sulfate, which are not native to the body, it is imperative to ask: Are vaccines making things worse, if not possibly the cause of many of our chronic ills?

Bad outcomes from vaccines are not unheard of, why? Citations of injurious inoculations in the medical literature go on forever and could fill volumes of books. But whether through vaccination or the introduction of any other synthetic chemical to our bodies, the disease process in the body does not begin with microbes, just with toxins. Anything foreign to the body disturbs its functions once it enters the system in any way.

Our bodies are being laid waste to by environmental contamination and deficient nutrition across the planet these days. It is no wonder, therefore, that we find many more activated forms of precursors present in the bodies of people who are presenting chronic symptoms of illness.

EIGHT

THE FLAW OF MODERN MEDICINE AND ITS INDUSTRIALIZATION

"Medicine, in fact, took a wrong turn when concentration on disease began to distract attention from the persons diseased."
THEODORE FOX

Many of the foundational arguments of modern medicine are based on weak assumptions about the behavior and processes of the body that have arisen from the unproven germ theory. One example is the popularized view of antigen-antibody complexes. Theoretically, such a complex is a molecule formed by an antigen bonding with an antibody. It is explained as a protective physiological response to foreign molecules. But there is common confusion about this and how the immune system, if in fact this system exists, actually works. Many health-care practitioners believe (and have been taught) the highly simplified notion that there is one type of antibody matching one type of antigen, and that these fit together like a lock and key. The truth is more sophisticated and fascinating.

In 1972, biologist Gerard Edelman, M.D., Ph.D., won the Nobel Prize in Physiology or Medicine for showing how antibodies can recognize an almost infinite range of invading antigens. (This honor was shared with biochemist Rodney R. Porter who determined the chemical structure of an antibody.) Edelman's insight, the principles of which resonated throughout his entire career, was based on variation and selection. He proved that what he called *antibodies* undergo a process of "evolution within the body" in order to match novel antigens. Crucially, he performed experiments on trying to discover the chemical structure of antibodies to support his idea.[1] Our bodies' natural capacity to address and remove new foreign substances they encounter make us strong beings.

The erroneous one antibody-one antigen theory bears a striking similarity to the one germ-one disease framework of the germ theory, does it not? Edelman's discovery has been oversimplified and reduced for the convenience of developing medical specialties, retaining scientific control, and capital gains.

During an interview in 1926, W. H. Manwaring, M.D., professor of bacteriology and experimental pathology at Leland Stanford University and twelfth president of the American Society of Immunologists, said, "Immunization to date has been based on the Ehrlich theory that the inoculation of disease products in subpathogenic doses creates antibodies, or, defending entities against any subsequent mass invasion. Not only is there no evidence of these so-called antibodies being formed, but there is ground for believing that the injected germ proteins hybridize with the body proteins to form new tribes, half-animal and half-human, whose characteristics and effects cannot be predicted... Even non-toxic bacterial substances sometimes hybridize with serum albumins to form specific poisons which continue to multiply, breed and cross-breed *ad infinitum*, doing untold harm as its reproductivity may continue while life lasts."[2]

Even to this day, the evidence about the nature of antibodies and our immune responses is sketchy. We don't fully understand the way antibodies work, being that they have only been observed under laboratory conditions and not in situations true to life.

When it comes to the incredible power of our body's regulatory processes, the confusion in mainstream thinking lies mostly in understanding that there is no such thing as an "immune system" *per se*. Terrain medicine views the body's main defense as its ability to detoxify itself. This is how the body self-regulates.

In the conventional medical paradigm, it is believed that a person encounters a microscopic organism, triggering many different cells to respond in a process known as *contracting a contagion*. After the body has provided itself with markers for identifying a problematic, invading organism, the body then stores the information about this organism so if ever the body is exposed to the same organism again, it will be impervious to the foreign organism. Every step of this sequence, from the notion of exposure to an invading organism to storing information in our "immune" systems is fictional, based on a small amount of variables that are accounted for only in the setting of a laboratory. The science doesn't truly explain what occurs in the natural world and the terrain of our bodies—in the wild, as it were.

In the field of propositional logic, it is recognized that some arguments are based on an affirmation of a fallacy. There are various names for this kind of argument. One is *abductive reasoning*. Other terms are *affirming the consequent* and *converse error*. The classic example of flawed reasoning is the paradigm of a broken lamp. While it may be true that a broken lamp causes a room to become dark, it is not true that a dark room implies the presence of a broken lamp. There may be no lamp or the lamp may also be switched off.

In mainstream science, we often find that the outcome of research assumes there is the equivalent of a "broken lamp." If a researcher goes into an experiment with the belief that microbes are contagious and does not challenge it, then they will never look for another explanation. Thus the results of their research are skewed before the study even begins.

This science only provides solutions for our health care needs that require us to employ aggressive, antagonistic treatments that are suppressive to our bodies' natural behavior. Billions are being generated by pharmacological companies each year. But if we could agree that there are no invaders or antibodies, then the industry of modern medicine would not need to devise their profitable solutions.

In addition to creating an opportunity for companies to invent and supply us with approaches to suppress symptoms, the germ theory enables companies to provide us with separate medications for each of the germs researchers tell us have invaded us. There is a single solution for every single invader. Unfortunately, the solutions we are being sold, based on a system of science built on the logical fallacy of germs, can produce serious side effects.

The solutions created by modern medicine in most cases are merely stopping symptoms. We live in a world of chronic illness, yet few medications offer true healing. What we need is to boost our bodies' true innate ability to restore their own balance, rather than rely on medications that often cause severe consequences to our health. If there are no invaders, as the terrain model shows, then what is called the immune system is really a system of restoration. This is why vaccines, for instance, are unnecessary. And beyond being unnecessary, they can be harmful.

A terrain doctor would never advocate for the use of a vaccine. Vaccinations are considered artificial tools for prevention of illness because scientists do not know how long the artificial reactionary measure lasts in the body. This is an unnecessary tool when there is not a full understanding of how the body works. Vaccinology is theoretical and most if not all test subjects are animals. A terrain doctor does not introduce substances to the body which the body's functions might interpret as toxins.

As of 2011, there had not been any correlative studies, either short-term or long-term, on the efficacy of preventing chronic illness or degenerative diseases with vaccines that were free from chemical contaminants.[3] Nor were correct or proper control experiments done to actually compare vaccines to a saline solution—serving as a placebo. I do not believe any have been done to date.

Well before the supposed COVID-19 pandemic, freelance reporter and former business editor of the newspaper *Financial Times of Deutschland* Torsten Engelbrecht and medical specialist in internal diseases Claus Köhnlein wrote the book *Virus Mania*, in which they assert that we should be wary of conventional science and its reliance on the science of antibodies—the use of antibody and PCR tests: "Such concerns only deepen when one considers that, besides freedom from liability, vaccine makers enjoy another little-known lucrative loophole: vaccines are the only pharmaceutical or medical products that do not need to be rigorously safety tested."[4]

One of the most significant things not being taken into account during the creation of vaccines is that scientists are messing around with super-microscopic organisms, like the precursors, which have not been measured in any manner prior to the development of these medicines. These could be present in the vaccine in a form that will elicit a massive clean-up in the body. Science unknowingly is exposing people to quantities of precursors combined with a humanmade substance, that may magnify the detoxification process of anyone who is injected. This could push the body of the person beyond the limits of its capabilities in an aggressive way (due to the introduction of the injection itself).

Vaccines are not an individualized form of medicine, as terrain medicine by definition is. Across the board, there are way too many variables to account for in order to inject any one person with a lab concoction that was not specifically formulated for that person and their current condition. This is a logical reason why we see such severely varying reactions from person to person after they receive the same type of injection.

As a terrain doctor, my belief is that the precursors are running off their last "program" of response to a specific cellular breakdown. After being injected, they follow that programming for a short time until they can adapt to the conditions in the new body.

There have been incidences when a recipient of the COVID-19 vaccines experienced myocarditis—inflammation of the heart muscle—blood clotting, anaphylaxis, Guillain-Barré syndrome, and severe lymphadenopathy. We really need not look too far to see how those who get that side effect were people who had a lot of prior wear and tear on that particular organ.

Outbreaks of avian flu in factory-farmed chickens, pigs, and cows have been widely reported by the news media in 2024. Yet these reports rarely depict the horrible conditions these animals live in. Nor do they discuss the various poisons used in the feed they are given to bulk up their muscles prior to slaughter, toxic chemicals like arsenic, synthetic hormones, excessive quantities of antibiotics, synthetic vitamins, and more. Despite the horrific, nonhygienic conditions in which they are raised, a virus is being blamed for the illnesses that arise. Millions of animals are impacted.

Chemicals Disrupt Our Internal Balance, Instead of Helping Us

In our society, we customarily take in a medicine to destroy or remove "hostile" infectious organisms. Because these critters are organic and adaptable in nature, the medicine has to be quite strong. In fact, this chemical-based medicine is usually so strong that it destroys the healthy surrounding tissues as well as the diseased tissues. So were we to look at a given "infection" site, we would find some healthy tissue, some destroyed tissue, some bacterial/fungal overgrowth, and the medicine, which is potentially toxic to both. Medicines, such as these are anti-life, destroying everything in their path. If you think about it, what does "antibiotic" actually mean when we parse the word? *Anti* means "against" and *biotic* means " living things." The name is accurate. Antibiotics destroy microorganisms like bacteria, and they also disrupt our cells and their processes—essentially being anti-human body!

After medication, the work the body has do is multiplied. Now, it must rid itself of three problem substances, along with the corrupted tissue that it was initially aiming to detoxify to restore its homeostasis. That seems like more work than just letting the body's system do its thing while supporting it with nutritious, unprocessed food, clean water, and rest.

Naturopathic doctors in the early twentieth century were already sounding the alarm about the insanity of the direction medicine was heading. This is nothing new. In 1913, in *Naturopath and Herald of Health*, for instance, R.D. Brandman writes: "Look at the Materia Medica of [allopathic medicine's] false and fatal system once more. If you could see it but one instant with clear vision and unbiased mind, you would recoil from it with horror. You would renounce and execrate it forever. What are its agents, its medicines, its remedies? Poisonous drugs, and destructive processes. Vaccines, toxines [sic], serums, scarifying, blistering, caustics, irritants, parasites, corrosives . . . all of the causes of disease known to the three kingdoms of nature. The effects of remedies are the phenomena of disease, and nothing else. We do indeed cure one disease by producing another."[5]

Some, like Bernard Lust, M.D., D.C., and N.D., who is considered the father of American naturopathy, went so far as to say: "Drugs can never cure a disease, but may cause a new one."[6]

As the new paradigm of germ and contagion embedded itself into mainstream society, the cries of natural doctors who promoted natural healing and opposed the germ contagion mythos were muffled by innovative industrial products that sold the idea of health in a bottle rather than promoting the health benefits of clean air, water, and healthy food. The industries that started to develop based on the dominance of the germ theory incorporated chemicals that suppress symptoms and further contributed to poisoning the health and terrain of both people and the environment—selling products for disinfection and sanitation, to name only two.

Because of Louis Pasteur's original reinforcement of the theory of contagion, an enormous industry for manufacturing drugs, antibiotics, vaccines, and many other germicides of all types developed. The fear of germs also became implanted in the human psyche and even became a phobia for many people.

As of this writing, this phobia has exerted its force so aggressively that it causes people to be haunted by the thought of spreading disease. They scrub, scour, and disinfect like crazy until their homes smell like hospitals. *Disinfecting*, *sanitizing*, and *antibacterial* are buzzwords used in sales pitches that catapulted billion-dollar industries to their success. Something as simple as a sneeze can drive some people into states of fear, leading them down the road of nervous exhaustion and the increased use of "cleansing" chemicals.

Though the management of these companies may have had good intentions, we now know, through many valid, reliable research studies, that the constant use of chemical disinfectants can only promote imbalance and creates "resistance" in many of the bacteria we see today. As these industries developed and lobbied in many government institutions, disease prevention soon became something sold in a product. Fluoride for tooth decay, preservatives in food storage, and even industrial oils were essentially promoted.

Other companies, such as those which make over-the-counter medications, also sell drugs to the medical industry like cocaine and morphine for pain relief, and mercury-based antiseptics like mercurochrome, instead of using natural choices like iodine and honey , for antisepsis. All these industries were able to profit and develop because of the constant fear of contagion. This constant fear of contagion was only reinforced by the fact that the living conditions in every city were deplorable.

Many writers of the early 1900s discussed ghettos in their works, mentioning the consequences of people living in crowded conditions without access to fresh air or clean water. It was in ghettos that most diseases flourished. Along with Upton Sinclair, who exposed corruption in government and business in the early twentieth century in his novels about the meatpacking industry, José Martí, who famously wrote about the struggle for Cuban independence from Spain, depicted this squalor in New York, where he lived later on, with the perspective of first-hand knowledge.

> *Their little dancing clothes disguise the children's sickly pallor and sunken cheeks! Health-giving air is in short supply where the workers live. Morgan, the former governor, has just left millions to theological societies and seminaries—but rather than working to force men to a faith in heaven, would it not be better to create that faith naturally by giving them faith in the earth? Morgan has*

> *also left considerable sums to homes where invalids, the elderly, children, and the poor are given assistance: couldn't he have left some money to help construct houses full of air and light?"*[7]

Edwin D. Morgan, who was governor of New York from 1859 to 1862, was known for his progressive values. But Martí did not believe his efforts went far enough. During this period, which coincided with the U.S. Civil War, hundreds of thousands, if not millions, of people were subjected to conditions that only supported diseases and toxicity. And as simple as it may be, today we know that one little yet important thing can alter the terrain, causing a person's body to shift out of its healthy state of homeostasis.

At the end of the nineteenth and beginning of the twentieth centuries, when the Industrial Revolution was well underway, factories were becoming commonplace. But there was little regulation or oversight of them yet, and conditions for workers were deplorable. industrialization was also significantly influencing the health of many members of the population.

One of the biggest industries to wreak havoc on human (and animal) health since that era has been the pesticide industry. In their book, *Circle of Poison*, environmental reporters David Weir and Mark Schapiro write: "Besides the widespread contamination of imported food, the overuse of hazardous pesticides has created a global race of insect pests that are resistant to pesticides. The number of pesticide-resistant insect species doubled in just twelve years—from 182 in 1965 to 364 in 1977, according to the UN Food and Agriculture Organization. So more and more pesticides—including new, more potent ones—are needed every year just to maintain present yields."[8]

The level to which people are exposed every day to noxious chemicals is immeasurable, especially in underdeveloped countries in warm climates, such as Mexico, Chile, and Guatemala, where much of the produce is grown that is imported by and feeds the people in wealthier nations like the United States. Though mainstream medicine wants to blame bacteria, fungi, and parasites for the diseases we experience, it doesn't take too much digging to find pesticides in everything that is eaten or touched. In terrain medicine, we recognize that our physical health is linked to our environment. Pesticides are known to diminish our health.

A person's day can begin with exposure to industrial chemicals, including even remnants of pharmaceutical drugs, that have gotten into the tap water they use to brush their teeth and make their coffee or tea. Chemicals in body care products, factory-processed foods, and the synthetic fibers (which most are derived from plastic) in our clothing can shift a good morning to a whole life nightmare of inflammation and pain.

In his book *The Hundred-Year Lie*, investigative reporter Randall Fitzgerald writes: "In 2001, scientists at the U.S. Center for Disease Control and Prevention in Atlanta surveyed 2400 people and searched for 148 specific toxic compounds in their blood and urine. Every single test subject contained dozens of these toxins. Children were found to be carrying more of the chemicals than adults, especially a class of chemicals called pyrethroids-found in most household pesticides—and phthalates, a group of chemicals distributed widely in plastics and cosmetics, primarily nail polish."[9] Phthalates are found in almost anything that carries a fragrance.

Two decades further along in our science, it is common knowledge that even things like cleaning supplies, building materials, office equipment, and air fresheners, all release chemicals, and long-term exposure to these can pose health risks to us. What is less commonly known is that they devastate the body's terrain. The toxic burdens many people carry are slowly breaking down the system within them. As cells in a person's body become toxic and die, constant production of bacteria and fungi from precursors is needed to clean up the mess. Annually, the Environmental Working Group releases a list for shoppers of the "Dirty Dozen" most pesticide-laden produce (visit EWG.org for up-to-date details).

Physician Richard Gerber, M.D., points out in his book *Vibrational Medicine:* "One problem with studying the adverse physiological effects of chemicals is the traditional scientist's inability to measure subtle changes in human beings. Certain chemicals may induce subtle abnormalities in behavior and mental alertness."[10]

Since the dawn of the microscope, science has tried to identify countless organisms isolated from their normal, natural environments in which they are found. The problem with doing that is in looking at an organism, any organism, outside of its familiar environment, it has a tendency to change itself and adapt. This is well documented, and truthfully, scientists should know better.

No matter what type of organism we are studying—whether a bacterium, a fungus, a mammal, or a tree—we cannot simply take the organism and plop it into a barren, sterilized environment, feed it "science-formulated" lab food, and think for one second that this living, breathing, and thinking organism will act the same exact way as it would in its natural environment. This is where the dogmatic, mechanistic scientific method has lost sight of the "holism" of studying microbes in their respective niches. Zoologists, botanists, and even mycologists (biologists who study fungi) understand how important and necessary an environment is to the organism they are studying. Pure lab isolation microbial growths inevitably will manifest in ways that do not truly replicate how they act and grow left to their own devices.

Having an erroneous picture of a microbe's necessities, like its food source and optimal conditions for thriving, devoid of humanmade toxic exposure, and even how it naturally dies, significantly alters the truth of how the microbe works inside the human body. Modern science only looks at microorganisms in this limited, not taking all the variables of negative stimuli into account, thus failing to fully appreciate all that is dynamically happening moment to moment in real life.

Microorganisms Help Us: Look at Nature

Removing a sample of bacteria from your throat, as your physician might do when suspecting a case of strep throat, and growing the strain in the medium of a Petri dish does not constitute a reliable scientific analysis of the organism. Remember how Dr. E.C. Rosenow at the Mayo Clinic moved strep to a new environment and watched it turn into staph and back again, proving it was the same organism. If bacteria are in your throat, I believe they are there to help restore the homeostasis of your throat, which has been disrupted somehow. It's appearance there is a clear signal that the tissue is in need of support.

If you have a sore throat, you would be better off finding out what bothered you, whether it was physical or emotional, eating foods that are simple, fresh, and nourishing, and getting lots of rest.

Our reliance on using chemicals in the study of microorganisms belittles the complexity of these amazing creatures that live in symbiosis with us. We would do well to shift our focus and study how microbes do all sorts of beneficial activities for animals and plants, as it does in all natural ecosystems all over the world.

Nature is a system in which the members mutually assist one another in thriving. There are organisms, like mycorrhiza, for instance, that help plants grow by synthesizing nitrogen for them. Mycorrhizas, symbiotic fungi found in the roots of plants, also help plants communicate. The main constituent of plant cell walls, cellulose is an insoluble, indigestible fiber for humans—found in vegetables and fruits—that aids us, when we need it, in processing waste better and prevents constipation.

Ruminant animals, such as cattle, sheep, antelopes, deer, and their relatives, contain a multitude of bacteria in their stomachs that break down the cellulose of all the plant material they eat. Humans do not have these bacteria or the multiple stomachs that these creatures have; nevertheless, we do have bacteria in our guts to help break down some of the foods we eat. Our gut microbiota produce hundreds of bioactive compounds, including essential nutrients, which play significant physiological roles in our bodies by supporting the fitness of symbiotic species and making sure the system maintains a flow and consistency of health. This mutualistic synergy can be seen in a multitude of niches, including the niches of animals, plants, and microorganisms.

Regardless of where they're found, there's one known consistency among all these microbes: Their jobs involve decomposition rather than the consumption of living cellular material. According to the latest research on the gut microbiota, there are tens of thousands, if not hundreds of thousands, of variations of microbes in the guts of the human population—everyone's gut contains a unique multitude—and modern science does not yet understand exactly what jobs they perform for us.[11]

PART II

THE BETTER WAY TO CREATE OPTIMAL HEALTH

NINE

□□□□□□□□

KEEPING THE BALANCE OF THE TERRAIN

"Freedom from fear, mastery of hygiene, and to never forget to treat the individual . . . to modify and adjust treatments to the individual case."
LOUISE LUST, N.D.

Hopefully, I've persuaded you by now that contagious microbes are not the root causes of disease, and you're ready to wholeheartedly embrace, or at least to test out, methods for improving and maintaining optimal wellness that are associated with the terrain model. Instead of focusing on a battle with malevolent entities, naturopathic terrain medicine, as it is practiced today, focuses on promoting balance, building optimal health by supporting the body in performing its natural functions through good nutrition, proper hygiene, getting adequate sleep and exercise, and detoxification, among other techniques. Supporting detoxification is especially beneficial, as it is the primary regulatory function of the body. When we support our tiny allies—the precursors in the various stages and forms of their existence—in cleansing our bodies of dead and decaying matter, our health improves.

To understand the terrain model is to understand that everything within our bodies is designed to establish and maintain balance down to the level of the cohesive dynamics in our cells, processes related to their growth, cellular division, and death, which occur with the aid of the precursors and the forms they turn into, such as bacteria and fungi. Everything we discussed in Part One. Optimal wellness in our terrain is characterized by establishing a dynamic balance between life and death, growth and decay. It is about creating synergy between the organs, and also synergy between the environments inside and outside the body.

The eastern philosophy of establishing a beneficial harmony of yin and yang (loosely, receptive/passive and active/directed forces) is similar to the terrain model of balanced health. In this instance, yang represents energy and growth, such as what might occur through consumption of food and strengthening your muscles by physical training; and yin represents rest, peace, and breaking things down, as might occur through sleep, meditation, and digestion.

Imbalances will show up in the body through its weakest link, whichever part of the body has the least resources it requires to function optimally. Deficient resources might be a lack of specific nutrients. Weaknesses might also be inherited predispositions of limited or skewed function.

And being that our nature as physical beings is electrical (or *energetic*, if you prefer that term), both in the way the human nervous system functions and in how our cells communicate, excessive exposure to electromagnetic fields (EMFs) can exacerbate susceptible nervous system imbalances as well, though these may not show up in classic disease form.

Over time, for example, an imbalance of the autonomic nervous system, which supplies nerves to the heart, skeletal muscles and glandular tissues, governs involuntary actions, such as hormone secretion and peristalsis; can show up as hypersensitivity, especially to energetic items like electrical machines and technology, or even to homeopathic remedies. Remedies such as homeopathic, have little to no physical presence as the potency of the remedies increase. Conventional medicine has yet to discover the principles behind the workings of homeopathy. What is known is that the more powerful remedies are extremely energetic, as opposed to material, and therefore it has been theorized that they become therapeutically altered when exposed to humanmade electromagnetic pollution.

If a person has a robust, balanced constitution, they will demonstrate physical, mental, and emotional resilience and appear to be glowing with health. Sure, small matters will always need to be addressed by them to serve the needs of their body, mind, and spirit and help them adapt to conditions, especially in cases of frequent exposure to toxins, including chemicals, emotional stressors, and the aforementioned EMFs, but rebalancing is always easiest for the person who catches it before an extreme imbalance depreciates resources which causes deeper physiological changes.

If someone becomes imbalanced, not only will they feel physical symptoms that correlate, but they also will be less mentally and emotionally resilient. They could feel irritable or become depressed and anxious, for example. Or their thinking may seem foggy.

According to the terrain model, there already has to be an underlying imbalance in an individual's body for them to become susceptible to an electrical or energetic substance and deem it harmful. Reimar Banis, M.D., contends that subconscious emotional problems arise from "substantial dysautonomia," a malfunction of the nervous system caused by an injury, poisoning, or chronic disease, like diabetes.[1] In plain language, this means that there already has to be a problem or imbalance that is interfering with bodily functions for certain substances to put a great deal of stress on the body.

That is not to say that something like 5G radio waves or Bluetooth earbuds would not be deleterious to the general well-being of any person. Just that, as the body responds to any other toxin, if it is working sufficiently and optimally, it will detoxify itself after the exposure. Banis also contends that 60–70 percent of people who claim hypersensitivity even to normal and natural things (because they tend to be wrought in their lives with emotional disturbance), become significantly less sensitive once the imbalance in their terrain is corrected.[2]

The term *hypersensitivity* has two meanings. First, that a minute quantity of a substance or a minute exposure to a stimulus, such as a noise or a flashing light, prompts a response. Second, that an exposure to a substance or stimulus provokes a response of exceptionally high magnitude. When someone has an outsized or hair-trigger response, we view them as being hypersensitive.

The good news is that hypersensitivity can be normalized to manageable sensitivity.

In his book *New Life Through Energy Healing*, Banis reinforces the idea central to terrain medicine that high-quality food, water, and air are important to our health. On an energetic basis, it is restorative to us, and balancing, for both our bodies and the foods and beverages we consume to have received adequate exposure to sunlight.[3] (He suggests an ideal exposure of fifteen to twenty minutes after cooking, but as everyone knows, the sun doesn't shine at night, so obviously this ideal is impossible to attain at dinnertime.) Sunlight reinforces the strength of our bioenergetic field and allows us to metabolize and consequently detoxify from exposure to toxins, including the negative, deleterious EMFs emitted by electronic devices.

Yin Dynamics and the "Soldiers" of the Terrain

Maintaining a balance of yin and yang energy applies to everything in our lives. Physically, this represents the balance of life and death, especially when it comes to the body's homeostatic processes of growth and decay. During gestation and shortly after we are born, we experience way more growth (yang) than decay (yin), so maintaining the body's homeostasis is rather simple then. That is why it is common for people to say, "When I was younger, I could do *this*, I could eat *that*, I could do *such and such* to my body, and everything would be fine. But now, my body cannot tolerate it."

As our bodies mature, the growth and decay dynamics even out. By middle age, it may be a bit harder to do certain activities without experiencing aches and pains afterward or causing ourselves some sort of mild to moderate discomfort. Once past that point, depending on a person's particular level of health, the scale balancing decay against growth tilts toward decay more than growth. Countermeasures must increase as we continue to age.

Funnily, in developed nations there is an opportunity for the body to be reinforced constantly, yet in most current industrial societies our choices reinforce decay because we are continuously introducing more toxins to our bodies. Eating packaged substances that their manufacturers pretend are food, which are stored in boxes and cans and saturated in preservatives, makes our bodies degenerate faster. If we eat junk food, we are bound to see a whole host of organisms in our bodies, sometimes new ones, as the precursors develop inside and around us, which transform into those microbes to help reduce the excessive amount of decay.

If you often see bacterial or fungal "infections" occurring in or on your body, this simply means there is more decay than growth going on inside you; these microorganisms are being called upon to do their job to remove the decay and reestablish your homeostasis. It is the body's job to ensure the correct equilibrium to support cellular growth rather than decay.

Yes, there will always be decay when we engage in physical activity, feel emotionally upset, or are stressed by turmoil, and so forth. There will even be decay that results from digestion and other normal metabolic functions—that's natural. But the idea of being a good caretaker of your body is for you to help reduce the amount of decomposition and cellular breakdown that is occurring, reduce the number of toxins you ingest that cause decay, reduce your exposure to preservatives and fake substances, diminish any vitamin deficiencies you have, live a less self-abusing lifestyle, and stop exposing your body to noxious poisons.

Bacteria, fungi, and even helminths should not be looked upon as parasites waiting to attack—as evil incarnate—but rather as supporters, helpers, and contributors making an effort to maintain the growth and balance of our inner universe, the kingdoms we call our bodies. They are the little "soldiers" on the front lines protecting, maintaining and preserving our optimal wellness that help our bodies do what needs to be done to restore their balance.

Interfering and not letting the precursors do their job of cleaning things up requires more energy on the body's part. Since disruption of health takes a toll that requires additional energy and nutrients to correct it, wouldn't it be better to have these organisms—these bacteria that we still call *germs*—do that work, and use their presence as a signal that we are not currently creating balance or health in our terrain but damaging ourselves? And then to take a good look to figure out how we are causing this damage and remedy it?

These microbes definitely support our yin-yang balance. Therefore, we should not destroy or try to remove them from our bodies. When they are present, it is a signal to remove toxins from our environment and reduce our exposure. If we are the ones exposing ourselves to toxins, we must stop adding more.

Supporting the Force of Life Within You

Many world cultures use the metaphor of light and dark to connote the balance between complementary opposite forces in our lives. As a terrain doctor, my approach to therapy is built on the same idea of the necessity for balance. Furthermore, I advocate that each of us embrace this approach in our daily self-care routines too.

Nineteenth-century French physiologist Claude Bernard viewed the force of growth in every cell as an expression of the ultimate life force. He believed this *bio force*, as he referred to it, represents a kind of intelligence. "In every living germ is a creative idea which develops and exhibits itself through organization. As long as a living being persists, it remains under the influence of the same creative vital force, and death comes when it can no longer express itself," he said.[4] Today, we conventionally would think of the intelligence driving a cell to function as it does as *genetic expression*, though that part of science, genetics, is still very limited in its understanding of inheritance and innate life force.

Essentially, what Bernard is saying in the remark above is that inside the pattern of life and death—right in the middle of push and pull, yin and yang—is vitality. The balance is maintained by the restorative mechanisms of homeostasis. When the equilibrium becomes erratic or disrupted, symptoms of detoxification ensue to sustain life.

Conventional medicine views signs of detoxification as different kinds of *diseases*. In terrain medicine, however, we hold the view that whenever the physiology and functioning of the cell or the life force within the cell is disrupted, the force of decay and death becomes stronger; and this state in the cellular environment signals the wonderful synergistic organisms we are calling precursors to morph into their next forms. These forms facilitate detoxification, then revert to their precursory state when it is done.

People often ask me why mainstream science doesn't share the same views as me. "Imagine this," I will say to them. When a scientist studies blood cells, the cells are analyzed out of context. They are taken out of the body and placed in a medium in which they don't normally exist, such as a Petri dish in the lab. But how are they nourished, oxygenated, and able to excrete there? Those are their normal functions.

The scientist might tell you—correctly—that blood extracted from the body is still "alive," because it is teeming with various organisms, enzymes, and such, which are slowly breaking the blood tissue down. But she would be incorrect in assuming that the cells display, on a physical level, the current standing of life in the body of the person from whom they were removed.

Science is deficient in its understanding of how the balance of life and death in the body is maintained. And using current conventional methods, scientists will never be able to measure the interaction of yin and yang (so to speak) in how the precursors are supporting life by removing damage from the body.

Contemporary terrain medicine uses diagnostic tools such as classical observation, thermography, and optical microscopy to study what is happening in people's bodies and practitioners draw their own conclusions from the evidence. These tools, if properly utilized, arrive at an understanding of the inner workings of the body in real time. This is important because a person's body needs to be evaluated contextually.

The main thrusts of terrain medicine are building up the body's strength, supporting its functions, and facilitating detoxification, all of which leads to the homeostatic regulation and the restoration of balance.

At some point, each of us has to take responsibility for our own wellness. We need to realize that even some foods and beverages we consume that are good for us in moderate quantities have the potential to become poisonous. Something as simple as water, adulterated and/or taken in bucketfuls, can create poisonous conditions in the body. These can cause havoc with our internal equilibrium, especially if the water is devoid of its natural components, like minerals.

By contrast, the well-known poison arsenic, which used to be used in pesticides but was banned in the United States in 2003, can actually be helpful to the body in minute quantities. If that sounds dangerous to you, please remember that, in fact, arsenic is naturally occurring in the body, and we do consume microscopic amounts of organic arsenic in our food—mainly in shellfish.[5] We are also exposed to inorganic arsenic in the air we breathe because it is a compound found in soil, rocks, and many building supplies, such as some pressure-treated woods, though exposure to these would always be considered toxic to the body.[6]

We ourselves are the determiners of what's poison for our bodies and what is helpful to them; although there are poisons, of course (predominately synthetic ones made in laboratories, even if derived from natural compounds) that will be toxic to us, no matter the amount of them we ingest. These are especially problematic for those of us who have slow or altered regulation or excretion in our bodies. The things that we need to stop exposing ourselves to include antibiotics, inoculations, and over-the-counter medications which suppress the communication that our precursors are trying to tell us about.

Something as benign as overindulgently eating a favorite food that makes us feel happy can potentially cause a disruption in our homeostasis. Day in and day out, we repeat activities that we think are "good for us," like exercising intensively or drinking a glass of red wine in the evening. But if we do not clearly understand the dynamic needs and ever-changing nature of our own body, we might be giving it something it actually does not need in the moment.

Initial signs of an imbalance are often subtle, therefore many of us do not heed the warnings we are given. Time passes, and sometime later on—for the sake of argument let's say ten years later—we have a more serious and painful problem because our indulgence and repetitive actions have destroyed certain processes of repair and disrupted the microflora in our gut. Due to our disrupted internal environment and the amount of time we have neglected to respond to the warnings, the initial signs of imbalance may have been amplified a multitude of times.

Nature likes balance, and when there's balance in the body and we add to it, we will not see any negative consequences. The rewards of balance that we reap are great health of the body and mind.

Changing our balance in any way is easy to see, especially when we are healthy. We merely have to pay attention to the signals that something is going off. By tending to these simple signs and symptoms early on, we can prevent the body from going into an extreme state of detoxification. If we ignore signs and symptoms, however, our body will show us in several ways. These ways become severely pronounced if the signs are perpetually ignored.

Of course, what I'm saying to you is traditional knowledge. Not a big secret. In 1908, naturopathic physician C.S. Carr, N.D., writing in the magazine *The Naturopath and Herald of Health*, said:

> *If a poisonous medicine is taken, at once the powers of nature are summoned to resist the intruder. What we call the operation of a drug is simply nature's method of getting rid of a foreign substance. What we call symptoms of disease are simply nature's efforts to restore the body to a normal condition. A quick pulse, a high temperature, rapid breathing, a dry skin or a moist skin; all these are the tactics which nature adopts to readjust the body to its environment.*[7]

Doctors in Carr's era did not rely on antibiotics like medical doctors do today because Andrew Fleming did not discover medicinal penicillin until 1928. Prior to their use, doctors of every tradition were trained to be observant of the body's innate mechanisms for restoring balance, and there were many therapies, some very simple, developed to do so.

TEN

□□□□□□□□

TERRAIN-MODEL THERAPEUTICS

"Terrain is shorthand for describing the uniqueness of an individual. We share experiences with others, but ultimately our terrain is ours alone. All aspects in our unique terrain bounce off of each other and interact with each other. Nothing acts alone."

HARVEY BIGELSEN, M.D.

This chapter offers a deeper discussion of the terrain model of health and healing. In it, you will learn about the different kinds of therapeutics traditional naturopathic doctors and health consultants use, and learn self-care considerations for use at home. What can alter the terrain of the body? How can we support the precursors that are engaged in the cycle of healing support for us? What are some of the normal functions of the body that microbes assist with? What bodily systems are most significant to this model of care? Answering these questions is essential to understand how to optimize your personal terrain.

What You Might Experience on a Visit to a Terrain Doctor

From the start, naturopathy, along with other types of holistic medicine, has adhered to the terrain model. Many who practiced it understood the great interlocking relationship between the body and the environment that surrounds the body. Some natural practitioners knew of the importance of the precursors (although they did not use this term). Once the germ theory became the dominant thinking of causation for illness, however, it caused many naturopaths and natural healers to forgo their understanding of our symbiotic relationship with everything in our terrain, including microbes.

Today, when visiting a practitioner who works based off of the terrain model, you will experience the fundamentals of nondiagnostic treatments. Since there is only balance or imbalance, therapies and remedies practitioners like me will suggest to you are applied with only one objective in mind, reestablishing your homeostasis. When my clients come to see me, I do my best to teach them to appreciate symbiosis and to help them understand whether or not their body's ability to self-regulate has been compromised in some way or their excretion has become limited.

The purpose of going to see a terrain doctor is fundamentally to receive education, guidance, and empowerment. In sessions with our patients, we are usually attempting to make our clients aware of the extraordinary and beautiful healing capacity of their own bodies. A well-versed doctor of terrain medicine teaches people the necessity of understanding, persistence, and experience when working with the body's inherent changes, and ultimately strives to give them tools and techniques with which the patients may reestablish a balanced terrain and achieve homeostasis after they have left the doctor's office.

The modalities that terrain practitioners use are designed to facilitate the healing responses within the human body. In utilizing various tools, such as isopathy and homeopathy, nutrition, and physical therapies like craniosacral therapy and massage, both practitioner and client must understand that the key to healing and reducing the outward symptoms of imbalance is detoxifying the body and replenishing its reserves of nutrients. This is how to support patients and their terrain.

Kinds of Therapeutics That Terrain-based Practitioners Use

The goal of traditional naturopathy, which is the basis of terrain medicine, is to physically, mentally, and emotionally help support the whole person, including precursors, in pursuit of optimal homeoregulation. *Homeoregulation* is the balanced and steady way the body optimally functions by way of digestion, absorption, assimilation, circulation, excretion, and so forth, to ensure flow and an efficient use of resources. This is a portmanteau of *homeostatic regulation*, a term coined by Walter Cannon to describe the innate and necessary mechanisms by which all life adapt to survive changes in the environment. During the patient's journey of homeoregulation, a practitioner may recommend a variety of therapeutic adjuncts to support them. Here are four that are most common.

Nutrition

The basis of all life, nutrition is a cornerstone of optimal health, serving not just as a source of energy but as a foundational element that influences every aspect of bodily function. The right nutrients support the body's complex regulatory processes, enhance the excretion functions, and promote overall well-being.

The body requires a variety of essential nutrients—minerals, vitamins, fatty acids, proteins, and carbohydrates—to function optimally. These nutrients support critical processes such as enzymatic reactions and cellular repair, to say the least. The foods we consume provide us with the energy we need for our daily activities and metabolic processes. The necessities of our material nature are such that we have to nourish ourselves; and given the numerous forms of animal and vegetable foods around the world that humans can make use of an assortment of diverse diets and ideas of what constitutes an appropriate diet has arisen. To consume food is a universal instinct, one that is influenced by the varied climates and landscapes people inhabit.

Because we have strayed from our perfect integration with nature and our society has become industrialized, chemical substances have been developed that imitate foods and beverages made from whole foods. Now that a number of generations have gone by in which our diets have consistently lacked the nutrients we need, to create good health in ourselves or to imbue good health in the physiology of future generations.

Your terrain-based practitioner will recommend nutritional solutions for you that are appropriate for your conditions and which will bolster your symbiotic relationship with the precursors living in your microbiome. By identifying imbalances and deficiencies, practitioners can recommend dietary changes that will facilitate healing and balance. Meeting your individual nutritional needs is paramount for your goal of optimizing your health. And remember, our nutritional requirements are not one-size-fits-all, as these are significantly influenced by a multitude of factors. Do not base your dietary choices on fads, but rather on the ancestral wisdom of nature. Dr. Weston Price taught that this is how we can ensure the terrain of the body is getting the correct support it needs for all its processes.

Herbs

Herbs have been used for millennia as a foundation of medicine and nutrition across cultures as well as the rest of the animal kingdom. Rich in bioactive compounds, herbs contribute to health in numerous ways.

The use of herbs dates back to ancient civilizations, including the Egyptians, Chinese, and Greeks. The ancient

Chinese, Korean, and Indian cultures employed herbs in their traditional medicine systems, all of which emphasized balance and harmony within the body through herbal formulations. Hippocrates, often referred to as the father of medicine, emphasized the use of natural substances, including herbs, in his clinical practice. His teachings laid the groundwork for western herbal medicine, which continued to evolve through the Middle Ages with the writings of herbalists like Hildegard von Bingen.

Many animals instinctively seek out certain plants when ill or injured. This behavior, known as *zoopharmacognosy*, illustrates their innate understanding of herbal remedies. For example, dogs may eat grass to induce vomiting or relieve gastrointestinal discomfort, while elephants have been observed consuming specific herbs to alleviate pain.

Contemporary studies have begun to validate many of the traditional uses of herbs, with research highlighting their pharmacological properties and potential therapeutic benefits. Natural health practitioners often emphasize the use of whole herbs rather than isolated compounds, recognizing that the full spectrum of phytochemicals in herbs works synergistically to enhance their effects.

Terrain-based practitioners utilize herbs the way the people in ancient and indigenous cultures traditionally do: with understanding of the synergy with nature. Herbs are not so much antimicrobial or destroyers of the life within, rather they support the rebalancing the body by way of increasing excretion, modulating processes or increasing efficiency of the regulatory systems. And in doing this, herbs beneficially alter the terrain by way of detoxifying it and causing down-regulation pleomorphism, which, in conventional terms, looks like microbe *destruction.*

Reassessing the value of herbs requires a shift in perspective from a narrow focus on their antimicrobial properties to a broader understanding of their role in promoting homeostasis and supporting the body's regulatory systems.

Homeopathy/Isopathy

Homeopathy was founded by German physician Samuel Hahnemann in the late eighteenth century. Hahnemann, dissatisfied with the prevailing medical practices of his time, began experimenting with various substances on himself. He observed that when he ingested small amounts of medicinal substances, he experienced symptoms similar to those caused by the diseases these substances were traditionally used to treat. This led him to formulate the principle of *similia similibus curentur* ("like cures like") that is the cornerstone of homeopathy. Next, Hahnemann began to experiment with highly diluted and potentized (shaken) versions of these substances, finding that they could effectively treat various ailments. His groundbreaking discoveries, published in *The Organon of the Medical Art* (1810), laid a foundation for the science of homeopathy, which continues to be practiced worldwide today.

The precise origins of the concept of *isopathy* remain somewhat elusive, with historical records offering glimpses of its emergence across different cultures; it is far older than homeopathy. Ancient texts reveal instances where substances believed to cause a disease were used, albeit in modified forms, to treat the symptoms. For example, the use of fox lungs to treat asthma, as documented by ancient medical figures like Dioscorides, Galen, and Serapion, hints at early applications of this principle. Additionally, the use of animal secretions to alleviate various ailments is well-documented in traditional medical systems across different world cultures.

In 1833, Herr Lux, a veterinary surgeon from Leipzig, published *The Isopathy of Contagions*, a book articulating the principle that infectious diseases contain within themselves the remedies for their own cure. This concept, while perhaps oversimplified, laid the foundation for the development of isopathic remedies.

It's crucial in our day and age to distinguish between true isopathic remedies and vaccinations. While both involve the introduction of biological materials into the body, vaccines typically contain numerous synthetic and humanmade substances alongside biological components of uncertain origin. By contrast, isopathic remedies utilize specifically defined biologicals derived from an organism or toxin associated with an illness.

Paracelsus, the renowned Renaissance physician and alchemist, occasionally alluded to the concept of isopathy in his writings. His disciple, Oswald Croll, further elaborated on these ideas, advocating for the use of healthy animal organs to treat corresponding diseases in humans. This approach, utilizing substances derived from healthy organisms, resonates with practices observed in various indigenous cultures worldwide.

Nineteenth-century physician Constantino Hering played a pivotal role in reviving the concept of isopathy in his century. He proposed the use of rabid dog saliva as a treatment for hydrophobia, a condition characterized by an extreme fear of water. This daring proposition, while controversial, echoed earlier ideas of utilizing the causative agent of a disease for its treatment. Hering further expanded on this concept, recognizing the potential therapeutic value of potentized extracts from healthy human tissues. He observed that these preparations exhibited a remarkable affinity for the corresponding organs within the human body.

How can we distinguish homeopathy from isopathy? While both therapeutics share a focus on stimulating the body's healing responses, they differ in their fundamental principles. Homeopathy, as outlined in Hahnemann's *Organon*, operates on the principle of similars, aka "like cures like." This means that substances that cause symptoms in a healthy individual can be used in highly diluted form to treat similar symptoms in a sick person who has a requisite profile of traits. Picking the correct remedy is an involved process that requires skill.

Isopathy operates on the principle of *equalia equalibus curentur* ("equals cure equals"). It utilizes substances derived from the very same organism or toxin that is presumed to be associated with the illness, albeit in highly diluted form.

Physical Therapy

An important aspect of health and life itself is the alignment and flow of fluids and energy through the physical body. Whether disruptions in this flow are avoided or corrected by the use of needles, like in acupuncture, the osteopathic manipulation of cerebral spinal fluid, or gentle massage that moves the lymph, the physical body benefits. The body is in constant need of realignment to ensure everything in it is moving as nature intended. Physical therapy keeps the bowels open, nerves firing, and much more, ensuring the most efficient and productive removal of waste and absorption of nutrients.

Osteopathic manipulative treatment (OMT). OMT is a hands-on approach used by osteopathic physicians (DOs) to diagnose and treat conditions affecting the musculoskeletal system. Founded by Andrew Taylor Still in 1874, the field of osteopathy emphasizes the interconnectedness of the body's systems and the importance of treating the whole person, not just the symptoms.

The emphasis of OMT is holistic. Its approach addresses the underlying causes of discomfort and dysfunction as well as symptoms. By focusing on the body's natural ability to heal itself, osteopaths aim to restore balance and improve overall health. Special techniques, such as stretching, pressure, and resistance, are used to alleviate pain, improve mobility, and promote proper flow of various fluids of the body and regulation.

Massage therapy. Massage is a manual technique that involves manipulating soft tissues (muscles and fascia mainly) to enhance relaxation, relieve tension, and improve circulation. With roots dating back to ancient civilizations in China, India, and Egypt, massage has a rich history of being used for both therapeutic and recreational purposes. Techniques like Swedish massage, developed in the nineteenth century, built upon these ancient traditions and laid the foundation for modern massage practices. Today, massage therapy is widely recognized for its numerous health benefits, including stress reduction, pain management, and improved recovery.

Chiropractic care. Chiropractic care, a field founded by Daniel David Palmer in 1895, focuses on diagnosing and treating mechanical disorders of the spine and musculoskeletal system, primarily through spinal manipulation. By restoring proper alignment of the spine, chiropractors aim to enhance nervous system function and improve overall body mechanics. Chiropractic adjustments can be effective in relieving various types of issues, including back pain, headaches, and joint discomfort.

Applied kinesiology. Applied kinesiology is a unique diagnostic and treatment method that utilizes muscle testing to assess the body's overall function. By evaluating muscle strength, practitioners can pinpoint areas of dysfunction or stress within the body. This approach allows for highly customized treatment plans that take into account physical and emotional factors contributing to the patient's health concerns. Applied kinesiology views the body from a holistic perspective, integrating various treatment modalities to address the root causes of imbalances.

Craniosacral therapy. Craniosacral therapy is a gentle, hands-on technique that focuses on the delicate membranes and cerebrospinal fluid surrounding the brain and spinal cord. By enhancing the flow of cerebrospinal fluid, this therapy can support nervous system function and alleviate conditions such as migraines and chronic pain.

Acupuncture and acupressure. Acupuncture and acupressure have been used for centuries to treat a wide range of conditions, including pain management, stress reduction, and digestive disorders. Acupuncture, with roots in ancient Chinese and Korean medicine, involves inserting thin needles into specific points along energy pathways known as *meridians.* Acupressure utilizes similar points but applies pressure instead of needles. Both techniques aim to balance the flow of qi (life energy) and restore harmony within the body.

Self-Care Considerations

The responsibility to our own health is of utmost importance because self-care prioritizes the particular activities that nurture and support our physical, mental, and emotional well-being as individuals. Engaging in self-care practices, at least simple ones to start, like eating food that is fresh and devoid of industrial processing, pesticides, and preservatives; breathing clean air; drinking fresh, clean mineralized water; getting sunlight every day; and doing some sort of physical activity consistently can support the regulatory and excretion systems of the body, creating the much-needed homeostasis for optimal adaptation to environmental stress.

The Most Significant Bodily Systems for Terrain Medicine

The human body has several systems dedicated to removing waste products and maintaining a stable internal environment. The kidneys, through the urinary system, filter blood and eliminate excess water, salts, and metabolic waste products as urine. The lungs, part of the respiratory system, expel carbon dioxide, a waste product of cellular respiration.

The liver, a vital organ, plays a crucial role in detoxification by processing and eliminating harmful substances. The intestines, part of the digestive system, eliminate undigested food and waste products through bowel movements. The skin plays a role in excretion through sweat, which removes excess water, salts, and some toxins.

Finally, the lymphatic system plays a crucial role in supporting the body's overall detoxification and waste removal processes through all of the aforementioned systems. It works closely with the transport of fluids, proteins, and various cells throughout the body. Lymph nodes filter lymph fluid, removing cellular debris, and other foreign substances. This helps to maintain a clean and healthy internal environment, most importantly supporting the work of other excretory organs like the kidneys, liver, and skin in eliminating waste products and toxins. These systems work in concert to maintain a healthy internal environment, ensuring proper bodily functions and overall well-being. These are the systems that are first analyzed by the terrain practitioner.

ELEVEN

□□□□□□□□

OVERCOMING MALNUTRITION CAUSED BY DEFICITS IN OUR FARMING PRACTICES

"He (man) has surrounded himself with all manner conditions, built himself an environment that reacts upon him every minute of his life, loads his digestive organs with the most ungodly foods, filling his body with poisons and when nature finally calls him to account he looks for a panacea that will relieve his suffering but at the same time to continue with his acquired habits of life."

BENEDICT LUST, N.D., D.O., D.C., M.D.

The most important development of resistance against toxic influence depends on receiving proper nutrition.

Think about it like this. A plant's resistance to parasites is just the plant being healthy. Parasites are not attracted to healthy organisms. Why? Because there is nothing in the healthy plant for the parasite to clean up. An interesting study was done by a scientist investigating the effect of soil health on plants. Those grown in poor-quality, naturally unfertilized soil would lose their leaves because of tomato worms. Intertwined within the vines were healthier plants that had been grown in a separate pot in fertilized soil, which did not have the same issue of destruction from the tomato worms. Their leaves were untouched, even though the same tomato worms could easily have crawled onto their healthy leaves, millimeters away.

A plant maintains health and vitality based on its nutritional intake, and it loses health and vitality in a way that welcomes organisms to break it down when it experiences a lack of adequate nutrition or the condition also known as malnutrition.

Parasites do not attack randomly; rather, they innately know either to help break down tissues that are already starting to decay or to remove the substances that are causing the deterioration. If we were to look closely at the origins of diseases like malaria, bubonic plague, and bronchitis, we would see that the presence of bacteria in all three cases is not an infectious cause but rather the 'cleanup crew' responding to an existing condition.

So, what does cause disease? The interplay of trauma, malnutrition, and excessive toxicity.

Malnutrition is the key that opens the doorway to a cycle of bodily responses known by medicine as *diseases.* Many researchers worldwide have emphasized that wherever they find tuberculosis and all sorts of degenerative diseases there is always malnutrition, too.

Toward the beginning of the twentieth century, Dr. Weston A. Price and others like him who were interested in factors contributing to our wellness arrived at the conclusion that disease occurs when the body lacks sufficient quantities of the nutrients it uses as its building blocks. To arrive at this insight, Price studied members of unindustrialized cultures that experienced no tuberculosis, which was more common in his era than ours, and no cancer and no heart disease of the sort that we are familiar in contemporary America, and he found a link between these conditions and the people's nutritional intake. Those less technologically advanced cultures were not riddled with the false foods we find on our supermarket shelves today. As a result, the people rarely got sick, their eyesight was sharp, their teeth and bones were strong, and their minds were clear well into their old age as well.

The practices of animal husbandry have always been an excellent source of insight into what might be happening to us when we eat our food. Those who raise pigs, cows, and chicken recognize that if a nutrient is lacking in any animal's diet, a disease of some sort will show up. In an address to the Florida Naturopathic Physicians Association, Dr. Royal Lee told a story about a farmer in New York State. This man made a contract with some hotels in his area to take their stale bread and rolls off their hands to use as hog and chicken feed.

> *His hogs had plenty of foods too, having the run of a large orchard with windfall apples. No scarcity of vegetation in*

the various by-product foods the farm offered. But the young pigs developed at only half the usual rate of growth and were subject to many diseases normally foreign to the pigs' species, particularly pneumonia. His Bradshaw pigs had small litters that were aborted, his hens began to lay eggs with irregularity, and the chicks hatched from them were so feeble that few survived. The only change that the farmer understood that he made was getting the stale bread and rolls and feeding them to his pigs and chickens. He then set up two test pens. The farmer put one group of pigs on the white bread and the other group back on whole grains and whole corn. In three months, there were pigs in one pen perfectly normal and healthy, and of course, the pigs in the other pen were quite sickly. This farmer was actually the Senator of New York, U.S. Senator W.P. Richardson of Goshen New York.

Senator Richardson himself said, "When I think of my experience in feeding pigs with the white bread leftovers of New York City's leading hotels, I am astonished at the indifference which white bread eaters manifest towards so many of their ailments. . . . The counterpart of these ailments on my pig farm, with all their distressing consequences, came upon me as a complete surprise. Had my pigs and chickens been eating nothing but white bread, I might have suspected the cause of the trouble before so much damage had been done; but they were rooting around and grubbing for themselves, getting lots of other food. I believe that the white bread consumed by them didn't amount more than half of what they ate, but it was certainly enough to cause a commotion at Goshen."[1]

One of the illnesses the pigs fed white bread presented with was pneumonia. Did the pigs "catch" pneumonia? No, they developed it after eating nutritionally deficient food. The development of pneumonia makes sense because, as their nutritional intake decreased, symptoms of pneumonia started to arise. As malnutrition increases in any animal's body, breakdowns start to happen.

In the early twentieth century, scientists learned that certain vitamins halt the production in the body of hormones that are usually present in the bodies of people with end-stage diseases, and they put two and two together and got four.

"No patient ever dies of a general infection, whether pneumonia or septicemia or even diphtheria," said Lee during his lecture, "if the normal vitamin C content was found in the body of the person."[2]

The Germans used to call diphtheria *fulminating scurvy*. Scurvy earned renown as a disease that sailors would get when they were aboard ship for months with no access to fresh foods, meats, fruit, and vegetables. What do we know about scurvy now? Scurvy is a vitamin C deficiency. That's why British seamen began eating foods rich in this vitamin, such as limes, and earned the monicker Limeys.

What is also known by science is that the toxins associated with diphtheria, the streptococcus and staphylococcus bacteria, cannot exist in the presence of vitamin C.

Pioneering vitamin C researcher Frederick Robert Klenner, M.D., was able to show how the bodies of peoples given vitamin C intravenously at high doses cleared not only diphtheria, but also streptococcus and staphylococcus, obviously altering the terrain of the body in a beneficial way.[3]

Other well-known illnesses, like polio and Ebola, have been studied enough to prove that people exhibit a "lack of contagiousness" if they are well supplied with vitamin C. In his book *Curing the Incurable*, Thomas Levy, M.D., writes: "Encountering the Ebola virus does not mean instant death. It is . . . highly unlikely that the Ebola virus could successfully sicken an individual with a good general nutritional status"[4]

In 1940, it was established by researchers T. Osborn and Josephine Gear that tuberculosis, which the World Health Organization lists as a "highly contagious disease," is something to which only mammals who lack the ability to synthesize their own vitamin C are susceptible.[5] Being that humans meet this criterion, we always need to make sure we are getting an adequate amount of vitamin C from the food we eat. Similar to animals, like the pigs from Lee's story, the foods that we consume need to have nutrients and vitality to support our wellbeing.

Many of the processed foods sold in supermarkets today have stabilizers added to them to increase their shelf life. Foods without additives spoil faster. But if your food does not break down on a shelf or get moldy quickly, how does that affect its nutritional content?

When you eat a piece of bread that does not grow mold in a couple of days, it lacks nutrients, which is well known since many companies add humanmade vitamins and minerals to compensate.

Another reason that I say so? Because intrinsic bacteria and fungi would be called to decompose nutrients in a fresh food. Their absence means that the food has been rendered lifeless by the manufacturers.

Here's the big problem. If you consume lifeless food, you are supporting the breakdown of your cells, which require you to consume nutrients that your body can use to maintain their functions, basically a steal-from-Peter-to-pay-Paul game. Many of the fruits and vegetables we consume (apart from those that are processed and lifeless) contain a limited supply of essential nutrition for us due to the poor levels of mineral salts and reduced enzymes in the soil we grow them in. In addition, many of us then destroy the little remaining nutrition in these ingredients by pasteurizing, microwaving, overcooking, and adding degenerated industrial oils to them.

Our Top Five Food Problems

It is essential to keep chemicals away from our farms. The meat and produce they supply for us and our families and communities are the building blocks of our bodies, and consuming poor-quality food made from ingredients containing toxic residue can prevent us from experiencing optimal health. This is true whether our food is sourced from plants or animals.

Germ theory has impacted the food supply adversely as farmers expend considerable effort on killing germs. The result of this is putting a strain on our whole society. Typically, crops are sprayed with pesticides and synthetic fertilizers. Nutrients are also deficient in them because the soil has become depleted through mismanagement of land and water resources. Livestock are treated with growth hormones and powerful antibiotics that destroy the microbes which life on Earth depends upon to sustain it.

In her book *Toxic Overload*, Paula Baillie-Hamilton, M.D., writes that we are now one of the most polluted species on the face of the planet and she basically infers that we are all so contaminated that, if we were cannibals, our meat would be banned from human consumption.[6]

Furthermore, the natural biological composition of both the plants and animals we eat is being physiologically altered in ways that make our bodies unable to digest and absorb their nutrients properly. Ignoring our synergy with nature as it originally existed frequently leads us to develop sensitivities that build into chronic ailments and interfere with the smooth functioning of our bodies.

The top five food problems disrupting our health based on conventional farming practices are:

- Pesticides.
- Synthetic crop fertilizers.
- Soil degradation and nutrient depletion through mismanagement.

- Livestock dosed with antibiotics and growth hormones.
- Large scale agricultural practices

Let's look at each of them in turn.

Pesticides

Since the inception of the practice of spraying on plants and animals to protect them from microorganisms, insects, and other critters, pesticides have caused havoc not only to the humans that consume the end products but also to the environment itself. Have we lost sight of the forewarning about the hazards of chemicals in early environmentalist Rachel Carson's book *Silent Spring*, published in 1962? Her book spurred a movement toward awareness of the impact of toxins in our food industry and put the chemical companies in an uproar. They didn't want anyone threatening their profits back in the day—and they don't today either. Despite the significant indications of deleteriousness of their use, pesticide use continues.

The first pesticides were largely derived from chemicals developed during World War I. One notable example is chlorinated hydrocarbons, which were initially used as chemical warfare agents. After that war, chlorinated insecticides were repurposed for agricultural use. Other toxic compounds, such as arsenic-based pesticides, were used before, during, and after that war, too. However, by the 1930s there was a significant shift toward synthetic pesticides, particularly DDT, which was in widespread use by the 1940s. By 1963, marine biologist and bestselling author Rachel Carson, testified before the U.S. Congress to urge for legislation against the use of DDT, which was banned. Even so many other synthetic pesticides are still being used today, sixty-plus years later.

Recently glyphosate, an organophosphate marketed under the brand name Roundup, was put under scrutiny for being linked by scientific research to non-Hodgkins lymphoma.[7] Its residue is found on corn, soy, wheat, cotton, canola, alfalfa, sugar beets, honey, and a variety of other fruits and vegetables grown on industrial farms in the United States. Slow, low dosing of a chemical like this one can cause endocrine disruption, reproductive deterioration, and severe changes in the gut mucosa that lead to malabsorption of nutrients and disordered excretion. Making severe changes in the gut microbiome has consequences for our health. Outcomes are similar for both humans and farm animals that eat tainted foods. Many other pesticides, even some that are used by large organic farms, will change the physiology of cell reproduction leading the person's body down the road to decomposition by the precursors rather than the maintenance of life.[8]

Synthetic Crop Fertilizers

Synthetic soil fertilizers, which also derived from petroleum, like many pesticides, were developed in the late nineteenth and early twentieth centuries, with the perception being that these were significant advancements for agriculture. Once superphosphates and ammonium sulfates became popular, crop production massively increased.

Although synthetic fertilizers may be a boon to producers, the environmental impacts have been substantial. Runoff of nutrients flowing into water bodies from fertilized fields is a form of contamination that leads to *eutrophication*, the accelerated growth of organisms, like algae, in water that deplete the oxygen content. This major disruption of the Earth's terrain affects the water supply of thousands, if not millions, of people in the regions of farms.

Having limited access to fresh water and constant intake of water contaminated by elevated nitrate levels is a severe problem. Contaminants can bioaccumulate in both humans and the marine life that we consume. Changes in our blood and the condition of our digestive tract, to the point where we contract cancer, are well-known adverse reactions to the consumption of contaminated groundwater.

Nitrous oxide that is heavily released into the air and soil disrupts various ecosystems as well as limiting the health and stored nutrient potential of the crops grown. Continuous use of nitrogen-based fertilizers can lower soil pH, leading to soil acidification and loss of soil fertility over time, harming various ecosystems including aquatic systems.

Soil Degradation and Nutrient Depletion Through Improper Management

Soil degradation and nutrient depletion are primarily caused by a combination of unsustainable, nonregenerative, nonorganic agricultural practices. Monocropping and excessive use of chemical fertilizers and pesticides strip the soil of its natural nutrients and disrupt microbial ecosystems. Additionally, poor land management practices, such as inadequate crop rotation and lack of cover crops, further exacerbate nutrient loss, soil erosion, and degradation. These factors all lead to the developments of crops that look fine on the outside, but yield poorly.

Nutrient-depleted plants are often weaker and in constant need of pesticides and fertilizers to stave off the pests that are trying to break them down further.

Livestock Dosed with Antibiotics and Growth Hormones

Feeding livestock nutrient-deficient feed can lead to a range of serious health issues and reduced productivity. Animals may experience vitamin and mineral deficiencies, resulting in weak bones, poor organ function, and reproductive problems. Young livestock often exhibit stunted growth and lower weight gain, while dairy cows may produce less nutritious milk or limited milk altogether.

Additionally, inadequate nutrition compromises livestock health, which leads to what would be assessed by conventional science as *infections*, causing farmers to give antibiotics and growth hormones for development and increased production of meat, eggs, and milk.

Growth hormones, administered to enhance growth rates and feed efficiency in livestock, lead to residues in animal products consumed by humans, potentially disrupting our endocrine and digestive functions. When humans consume cattle, poultry, or dairy products containing the residue of an antibiotic, this contributes to severe deterioration in the balance of the microbiome. Proper maintenance of cellular construction within the body degrades, adding to long-term effects of degenerative diseases and increased cancer risks.

Large-Scale Agricultural Practices

The practices associated with large-scale agriculture compromise the health of ecosystems, animals, and human populations. The intensive use of chemical fertilizers and pesticides to maintain or increase production of crops leads to a severe deterioration of soil, water, and air in the vicinity of farms. Similarly, livestock confined in poor conditions contribute to the degradation of the surrounding environment through their excrement, which is toxic due to illness and medication. This pollution sickens wildlife and poses health risks to humans, including risks of increased rates of cancer and other diseases linked to chemical exposure.

Large-scale farming significantly reduces or entirely destroys biodiversity in plants and animals primarily through monoculture practices, where vast expanses of land are devoted to a single crop species. This lack of crop diversity diminishes the variety of plants in the ecosystem, making it more riddled with pests and diseases, which in turn encourage increased pesticide use. The resulting chemical inputs can harm nontarget species, including beneficial insects, like bees and other pollinators, birds, and soil organisms, further disrupting ecological balance.

For livestock, large-scale operations often prioritize production over animal welfare, leading to overcrowded and unsanitary conditions that can foster what is perceived as disease outbreaks, when in actuality, it is poisoning. This impacts our food safety.

Through causing chemical exposure, water contamination, and ecosystem destruction, while producing low-quality food, large-scale agricultural practices are contributing to the disturbance in the homeostasis of animals, plants, and humans alike.

Ways to Overcome the Problems Within Our Agricultural System

"The threat to our health comes not only from individual chemicals but from the total chemical load we are sustaining and the interactions of the hundreds of chemicals stored in our tissues. Certain chemicals in combination become thousands of times more toxic than anyone acting alone."[9] To overcome the deleterious effects of large-scale, chemically oriented agricultural practices, a shift toward sustainable farming methods is essential. Implementing practices such as crop rotation, cover cropping, and agroforestry can enhance soil health and reduce the need for chemical fertilizers. When they are utilized, these methods improve soil structure, increase organic matter, and promote biodiversity—factors which, in turn, support the development of healthier ecosystems capable of naturally regulating pests and diseases.

In addition to sustainable farming, several other environmentally friendly farming styles are known to contribute positively to ecological health. For example, there is **organic farming,** which avoids synthetic fertilizers and pesticides, but utilizes natural inputs and the rotation of crops from planting season to planting season to enhance soil fertility and promote biodiversity.

Permaculture focuses on designing agricultural systems that mimic natural ecosystems, emphasizing biodiversity and resource efficiency.

Agroecology integrates ecological principles with agricultural practices, fostering local knowledge and community involvement while maintaining soil health.

Regenerative agriculture aims to restore previously damaged ecosystems through practices like cover cropping, reduced tillage, and enhancing soil vitality.

Biodynamic farming incorporates organic practices with holistic management techniques, treating the farm as a self-sustaining organism.

Lastly, **conservation agriculture** emphasizes minimal soil disturbance and crop rotation to improve soil health and reduce erosion. Collectively, these farming styles work to protect the environment while ensuring food security and resilience.

Promoting alternative livestock management practices, including the understanding that certain germs are present *because of* the negative consequences of chemicals and poor agricultural conditions and not the causes of disease, can significantly reduce the reliance on antibiotics and improve animal welfare.

Implementing rotational grazing and providing environments enriched with balanced microbiota can enhance the health and productivity of livestock while reducing symptoms of disease prevalence.

Encouraging smaller, local and organic food systems to be incorporated could help every town and city create a more resilient agricultural landscape that prioritizes quality over quantity and reduces the pressure to produce high yields at the expense of health.

Policymaking that supports sustainable practices and providing incentives to farmers who adopt ecofriendly methods may play a crucial role in transforming the agricultural sector. However, education on the existence and function of precursors and the interweaving of people and the environments they live in will be necessary. By prioritizing farming practices that are nurturing to the growth and wellbeing of the whole planet, we can address soil degradation, air pollution, and the negative impacts of chemical dependence, ultimately leading to healthier food systems and improved public health.

For the sake of your own health and the health of your family and community, take steps to ensure that your food, water, and air are as clean as possible. Purchase from the farms and companies that keep sustainability and clean living in mind. Throwing your support to smaller farms that are environmentally conscious could save you extra trips to see a health-care practitioner who will invariably tell you that you are toxic, filled to the brim with an accumulation of poisons from all sorts of exposure.

Ultimately, there is only one choice for your health. That is to follow the rules of nature: Consume clean water, clean air, and fresh, unadulterated, "clean" food, and be sure to expose your skin to sunlight whenever possible. The ideal "dosage" is twenty minutes over 20 percent of the body.

The Top Five Health Problems That Fake and Toxic Foods Are Causing

Although the processing of food by salting, pickling, and drying it is a technique that is thousands of years old, when we refer to *processing* these days, we are referring to the techniques of industrial food processing, which generally started being used in the late nineteenth century. These methods include chemical fermentation and smoking, artificial preservation, refinement of ingredients, and the development of convenience foods.

Because of all this, we now have foods in our pantries that, scarily enough, may keep indefinitely. Microorganisms do not even break such foodstuffs down, which means we really should not be eating them. Nutrition comes from the breakdown of food into absorbable molecules—from *metabolism.* Unfortunately, the thought that "because processed food lasts forever we cannot metabolize it" does not cross the minds of many people, so they continue to consume these foods causing many if not all the ails they are experiencing.

Health Problem 1. Nutritional deficiency. Processed, artificial, nutrient-depleted foods are stripped of anything real that the body requires, such as minerals, fatty acids, enzymes—basically their life-giving elements. Many processed, industrially produced foods are designed to be shelf-stable and hyperpalatable by relying heavily on added sugars, artificial flavorings, and a mix of ingredients that many of us normally would not choose to consume on their own merits if it were not for factory processing, their availability in grocery stores, and their low prices. The consumption of processed foods can create a cycle of poor dietary habits that exacerbate nutrient deficiencies.

Although these fake foods may feel satiating as they are consumed, their low nutritional value causes us to overeat them because they do not fulfill our bodies' nutrient requirements. Over time, this results in nutritional deficiencies and sickness that manifests initially as symptoms of colds and infections, and further down the line as chronic, degenerative disorders. Symptoms that are interpreted by conventional doctors as evidence of bacterial or fungal infections are merely evidence of the deconstruction of a decaying system due to its lack of nourishment.

Our bones and teeth are tissues that consist of an elastic protein matrix which requires certain nutrients to sustain it. But sadly, processed meats, instant foods, and ultra-pasteurized dairy products are devoid of anything that contributes to the well-being of bones and teeth. And in fact, such foods can harm teeth because they will strip the body of the needed minerals and proteins.

Health Problem 2. Malabsorption. Mass-produced foods can contribute to malabsorption of nutrients and mucosal membrane irritation through several mechanisms. Many contain additives, preservatives, and other artificial ingredients that can disrupt the gut microbiome. When the balance of the bacteria is altered, it can lead to dysregulation of the terrain of the gut, and diminish the integrity of the intestinal barrier, a condition that impairs nutrient absorption.

Additionally, certain compounds found in processed foods, such as rancid industrial oils and high levels of refined sugar, can cause congestion and irritation. Conditions like leaky gut syndrome, ulcerative colitis, and the like, which occur when the intestinal barrier becomes permeable, allow undigested food particles and toxins to enter the bloodstream. As the irritation of the mucosal membranes persists and more toxins leak into the system, the excretory systems, including the kidneys and liver, which are responsible for filtering toxins and waste products from the body, will eventually be compromised.

The ongoing buildup of toxins that have not been eliminated along with the malabsorption of essential nutrients can lead to a massive lack of resources. As the body draws from its already limited stores of nutrients this will further aggravate existing nutrient deficiencies. Eventually, the starvation of the cells can lead to cascading die off and increased microbial cleanup, which looks like a massive infection and an exhausted body in a state of systemic decomposition.

Health Problem 3. Toxicity. Artificially manipulated foods can cause toxicity in the body and brain through several pathways. Certain food dyes and preservatives, for example, have been linked to adverse health effects, including neurotoxicity, which can disrupt normal brain function and contribute to behavioral issues or cognitive decline. That is what a toxin is: a substance that interferes with normal cellular function. The problem is that as the system starts to reduce its capability of being able to remove these noxious substances, the degree of severity of their impact on the body increases. As these toxic compounds accumulate, they will begin to impact the function of all the organs.

Overload can eventually affect the whole system, especially the aspects of it that manage waste disposal. Excess chemical and nutrient elimination can disrupt the balance of the terrain and disrupt the microorganisms required for proper waste breakdown. The terrain of a toxically overloaded body eventually changes to a point where the precursors become exhausted.

Health Problem 4. Chronic inflammatory responses. Artificially created foods can trigger chronic inflammatory responses primarily through their toxic composition. The body reacts poorly to these substances when they are lurking in the system. Inflammation is a crucial biological response that helps protect the body from harm. By increasing blood, lymph, and oxygen flow to a damaged area, inflammation promotes the regeneration of cells and the release of essential growth factors in the tissue. But when there are repetitive assaults coming from the consumption of pesticides, preservatives, and hyper-processed ingredients, the inflammatory process is forced to continue endlessly. And that creates incredible discomfort and begins to deplete the body's protective resources.

Many of the substances added to processed foods have not had rigorous long-term studies done to show their lack of effect when these substances are consumed repetitively and in massive amounts. Those which are not metabolized or easily eliminated may incite the body to maintain use of its protective mechanisms constantly. This includes relying on the precursors, in their stronger stages, to try to remove or sequester offending materials so that they won't be able to impact the whole body. Isolated locations of inflammation in the body are usually indications of toxic buildup. In this way, the precursors and the inflammation are acting as one in the same, protection and prevention from total breakdown.

Health Problem 5. Reproductive and developmental issues. Many of the processed, chemically laden foods contain endocrine-disrupting chemicals, such as phthalates, bisphenol A (BPA), and certain artificial additives, which can interfere (at the very least) with a woman's ability to ovulate or conceive and with a man's libido and ability to produce sperm. In addition to direct reproductive impacts, the preservatives and low nutritional value in processed foods can contribute to obesity and metabolic disorders.

Constantly being exposed to the additives in the fake foods can complicate reproductive health and fetal development. Maternal nutrition during pregnancy is critically important for the healthy development of a fetus and early health of an infant once it's born. Exposure to any of the toxic preservatives, chemicals, and artificial ingredients so common in our food supply may lead to complications such as low birth weight, developmental delays, and an increased risk of needing health-care interventions at a very early stage of life.

The impact of the interference of these items on the terrain of a developing human has not been studied enough to allow them to be consumed safely in any amount during pregnancy.

TWELVE

□□□□□□□□

DETOXIFICATION AND REDUCING THE BODY'S WORKLOAD

"The environment for one individual is never the same at any two moments in time and is constantly changing. Hence, symptoms will unpredictably change, and even things that once caused reactions may not cause a reaction on another day because the total load is never the same. For example, the office paint will bother someone more after a night of alcoholic drinks or a night in a smokey bar . . . The detox system needs time each day to catch up."
SHERRY A. ROGERS, M.D.

Precursors in all their different forms are part of the cycle of life in Earth's ecosystems, including the micro ecosystem that is the individual human body. The underlying reason for precursors to pleomorph into bacteria and fungi in the human body is to hasten the body's removal of decaying cells and digestive waste, and to aid in its various detoxification processes. The human body naturally rebalances its terrain using whichever resources are at its disposal, but if your body cannot keep up with the metabolic work of breaking things down and eliminating them, then you will begin to feel toxic. This is the sick sensation you would get from overeating meals, drinking alcohol until you're tipsy or smashed (in-*toxic*-ated), breathing noxious fumes, and much more.

In this chapter, I will explain how to support your body in rebalancing through its natural detoxification processes. I will include mention of additions you can take to help repair the function and physiology of the stomach, intestines, liver, kidneys, pancreas, and gall bladder in their functions. And I will explain how essential rest and recuperation are for proper homeostasis. Finally, because of conventional medical thought, I will also remind you that taking medications to kill germs is not warranted. Not only can medication be toxic, but it can sometimes be deadly.

Intoxication by Means of the Substances We Ingest

Intoxicants are taken by many in the name of medicine and health. Though these are sold freely and consumed even more freely, they afford the body no advantage, despite the temporary powers of strength and euphoria they elicit. From studies and experience in practice, I am convinced that all of these additives in our diet eventually cause weakness, depression, and premature aging, and that many, if not all, of these substances directly or indirectly alter various tissues in the body to deterioration, which is contrary to the nutritive, life-giving power of natural food. To advise or encourage the use of any of these for anyone is in direct opposition to nature's laws within our body. This is in a way an abuse to preservation of our health. Below is a list, though not exhaustive, of items that will stress and tire your bodily systems.

Toxins in foods. Refined sugar, artificial sweeteners and colorings, preservatives, ill-prepared foods, instant foods, fake flavorings, thickeners like acrylamide, synthetic vitamin additives that you might find in products labeled as "enriched," synthetically derived vitamins and mineral supplements, margarine, trans fats in fried foods, heavy metals, and pesticide residue, among other things. In addition, food may be contaminated by nonstick coating on cookware, plastic wrap, and plastic food containers.

Toxins in beverages. Caffeine, refined sugar, alcohol, artificial sweeteners and colorings, fake flavorings, preservatives, heavy metals, pesticide residue, bisphenol-A (BPA) found in many plastic bottles, formaldehyde, and fluoride, among other things.

Other toxins. Tetrahydrocannabinol (THC), the active ingredient in marijuana, e-cigarettes, heavy metals, home furnishing chemicals, like formaldehyde, clothing chemicals, pesticide residues in fabrics and wood, household products and their fumes, phthalates (found in some cosmetics, shampoo, nail polish, skin cleanser, aftershave lotion, and hair spray, perfumes, laundry detergents and even newly made clothing), fumes from heated plastics, volatile organic compounds (VOC) from paints and cleaning products, carbon monoxide (from furnaces or boilers, vehicle exhaust, clothes dryers, fireplaces, gas stoves and ovens, and more), and so many more.

It is here we should remember, especially from the previous chapters, that it is not the toxic substance that is so much the problem, but rather it is the person's reaction to, and stabilization following, the toxic exposure. The stronger the regulatory and excretory systems in your body, the better your body will be able to handle the metabolizing of different substances as it breaks them down and excretes them. This is why it is most important to ensure the maintenance and optimal performance of the modes of detoxification with the least amount of effort.

Natural Detox Systems of the Human Body

Many of the diseases and symptoms of illness that we see today are reactions to the environment, indications of toxicity. Most people live in environments that are swimming in toxicity. We are supplied medicines full of toxins, foods full of chemicals, air full of noxious substances, and even water full of pollutants. If at any point the natural mode by which the body removes these deleterious substances becomes faulty in any way, it builds up and creates symptoms.

Initially in life, a person's body is quite efficient in removing harmful substances. But over time, especially if fueled incorrectly, overloaded by stressors, or nourishment has been neglected, the toxins will build up.

The natural detoxification systems of your body include defecation, urination, breathing, and skin release (through sweating, oil production, and more). These are essential to the equilibrium between growth and decomposition. The body operates on the principle of homeostasis, which is a form of maintenance within the range necessary to stay alive.

In my naturopathic practice, after helping people reduce their exposure to toxins through their food, beverages, and households, they find that homeostasis is easily restored. As you become healthier, your body's rejection of toxins will become less apparent to you because your body will become more efficient. As your excretion avenues become more efficient, the paths to eliminate the toxins will be faster and less noticeable.

The Four Levels of Elimination

There are four methods of elimination that the human body uses to get rid of its own waste (such as the byproducts of metabolism and the turnover of dead cells) and toxins. When there is interference or suppression on any of the easier levels, the body will resort to using the next level of elimination in order to get the job done. If you perceive a symptom in any of your physiological systems, it is a sign that your body is doing its natural work of elimination of something that is no longer (or never was) useful to it.

The four levels of elimination are all reactions to substances that are unwanted.

Level 1. Primary reactions. The first level of removal of toxins encompasses substances that are produced as waste during the performance of normal bodily functions, such as digestion and breathing. These functions can happen in varying degrees of success depending on the particular body: its age, the synergy of its organs, and how optimal the condition of its lungs, skin, intestines, kidneys, or liver. If a person is well nourished, then little effort is required for the body to excrete anything successfully. This is the most optimal and supreme form of elimination. It is also the most optimal experience of health.

Level 2. Secondary reactions. This level of removal of toxins relates to bacterial production and, in some cases, to fungal production. Manufacturing these organisms in the body is necessary when cellular decay or excretion is occurring at a very high level and/or the normal methods of excretion are being disturbed in some way, either by internal stimulus or external interference. Examples of this include what conventional science labels as infections, especially those that occur prior to the involvement of the so-called immune system.

Symptoms of secondary reactions include diarrhea, congestion, runny nose, coughing, sneezing, and the like. Initial cellular degeneration can be caused by lowered vitality due to overworking, excessive eating and drinking, drug and alcohol consumption, and encountering emotional or psychological stressors, among other things. As these behaviors and experiences increase, so does waste material in the body. A secondary reaction, along with any other toxin and a lack of proper nourishment, leads the body down the path of utilizing more extreme physiological detoxification measures.

Inheritance of poor physiological or psychological responses and other chronic happenings and suppression of the acute response can certainly lead the body down the path to the stronger, tertiary reaction—and possibly farther.

Level 3. Tertiary reactions. The third and more aggressive level of elimination involves the many diverse types of blood and lymph, such as white blood cells and platelets. If microorganisms, such as our bacteria that are playing a role in elimination of debris in the body, become overwhelmed, then white blood cells (leukocytes) are activated. These cells will help create space for further consumption of both the debris and any dying microorganisms. Meanwhile, the platelets—seen as tiny fragments of blood cells, play a role in blood clotting and the repair of damaged tissues—create a web of support for the bacteria and leukocytes. Platelets also communicate with the body's various cells within areas of trauma to act in cooperation and create zones of sequestered irritation or stagnation to be addressed later by the body.

Whenever there is toxic overload or damage to some tissue, the body's production of different types of blood cells increases. An urgent need for cell production calls for an increased use of the body's nutrient stores, especially the stores of nutrients held by important organs, such as the adrenal, thymus, and thyroid glands, the spleen, the bone marrow, and the liver.

Several organs—of different types—take part in removing unusable material from the body's tissues along with excess dead or dying microorganisms and white blood cells. The lymphatic system, for instance, is used to cleanse an area of tissue, which is a process similar to spraying down a sidewalk after many dead leaves have fallen and been raked up. The lungs help remove some of the "junk," while the liver and kidneys utilize their own respective avenues of evacuation. Both of these organs serve as filters and the debris they collect ends up being released in our urine and stools.

Tertiary reactions represent the inflammatory stage of excretion. Inflammation, as you've learned in this book, is a beneficial and natural mechanism whereby the body works synergistically with microorganisms in the terrain to attend to breaking down and removing unwanted material. Symptoms of this level of elimination include high levels of neutrophils and/or basophils in the bloodstream (more technical names for particular white blood cells), enlargement of the liver or spleen, and more.

Although inflammation is often seen as a negative experience, because it is physically uncomfortable, it is actually a very helpful and extremely necessary bodily response. Many people, though, get stuck in a loop of constant inflammation and excretion. If they are ignorant of what to do, instead of helping themselves with natural means, such as improving their diet, reducing their exposure to chemicals, or increasing their use of helpful modalities like chiropractic care, supplementation with herbs, or resting, they may wind up taking antibiotics and anti-inflammatory medication that compounds their trouble. New exposures could keep them cycling through reactions on this level.

Level 4. Quaternary reactions. This most intense, exhaustive level of removal of toxins involves the expulsion of dead tissue and debris. Symptoms of this order of reaction include, but are not limited to tumor production, limited or failed production of specialized blood cells, a change in the function of one or more organs to the point of its deterioration, and the almost complete reduction of regular cellular functioning.

To aid in the expulsion of toxic materials, the precursors are instigated to reproduce themselves in massive quantities, creating storms of precursors prepared to do whatever it takes to support the system. A quaternary reaction is the strongest reaction that we have to toxic material in the body, and we only see symptoms of this type of reaction if someone has been injected with a deadly poison—either by natural means (such as a bee sting or snake bite) or by medical means (such as a vaccination or an IV drip).

When the body is having this type of massive adverse reaction, the body will continue increasing its efforts to push out the cells destroyed by the poisons until it becomes much more nutritionally deficient.

Each level of elimination described above requires more effort and nutrition to be successful than the level before it did. If the body is already deficient before a stimulus, or if the frequency with which a person's body must excrete damaged cells and toxins occurs at the highest levels for a while, the body's cycling through the four levels of elimination becomes chronic. Chronic toxicity requires it to draw repeatedly on the same repair mechanisms until the organs involved in these functions reach exhaustion.

You can see this type of exhaustion occurring in people struggling with pneumonia who are becoming increasingly septic, for example. Or in people who cycle on and off of antibiotics, attempting to cure chronic "infections." Chronic arthritis is another very good example of how the body can cycle through the first, second, and third levels of elimination reaction before expressing a fourth-level reaction.

Common Stressors That Factor into the Interactions of Precursors with the Human Body

A foundational understanding of proper healthcare lies in recognizing the effect of stressors on the terrain of the body. Various factors levy the body's processes, including mental stress, compounding one problem into many. But in general, our nutritional habits play the most critical role in the ability of our bodies and minds to withstand the onslaught of stressors. Nutritional deficiencies and overreliance on processed foods can weaken our bodies' ability to maintain balance. This creates an internal environment that makes us more susceptible to toxicity. For a weakened body, exposure to environmental toxins, such as pollutants and chemicals, can overwhelm the body's detoxification systems, leading to an accumulation of harmful substances. We naturally begin experiencing symptoms of detoxification, which make us feel sick.

Toxicity is not the only stressor we may face. **Postural misalignments and physical malformations** are also stressors that can disrupt our physiological functions.

Mental and emotional stressors, such as daily challenges and relationship problems, among other things, can cause us worry, grief, anxiety, and depression, taking a toll on our overall health. **Unresolved trauma** exerts a profound impact on both our physical and mental well-being.

Social stressors, like isolation, discrimination, bullying, and lack of human support, can also have a profound impact. These stressors singularly or combined can create significant distress and negatively affect our overall mental well-being.

This set of stressors can be broadly categorized into two main groups: physical stressors and lifestyle stressors. **Physical stressors** include injuries, illnesses, surgeries, chronic pain conditions, and malnutrition. These can place a significant burden on the body's systems, leading to stress responses. **Lifestyle stressors,** such as poor diet, lack of sleep, excessive caffeine or alcohol consumption, and lack of exercise, also contribute significantly to physical stress. These unhealthy habits can disrupt bodily functions, weaken the excretion systems, and increase a display of various health problems.

Environmental stressors encompass a range of factors that can significantly impact human health. These include physical factors, such as noise and air pollution, extreme variations of temperatures, and lack of access to green spaces. Natural disasters, like earthquakes and floods, can also cause significant physical and emotional trauma. Chemical exposure to pesticides, herbicides, and industrial pollutants poses the most health risks, especially when the air, the food, and the water are highly contaminated.

Light pollution from exposure to excessive artificial light along with many chemicals from artificial living spaces stresses us out, too. In addition, exposure to electro-magnetic fields (EMFs) from sources like cell phones and power lines have been known to cause negative health effects in those who lack homeostasis.

The Far-Reaching Implications of Adhering to the Germ Lie

The magnitude with which germ theory has perversely invaded almost every single type of industry is enormous. In medicine, this means having the one disease leads to one treatment, or a certain group of approved treatments for one disease pattern. The treatments are designed by the medical industry to implement their control over us. A variation of any disease becomes known as a "new" disease, creating new profit opportunities for an overinflated industry.

Other industries that have prospered from adherence to germ theory are the sanitation industry, the processed food industry, and agriculture. Any companies that profit from killing germs that we might breathe in the air or contact through our skin depend on our continued belief in the germ model for their success. Sterility and decontamination companies are others.

Most sinister, from my point of view, is how the food industry has loaded our consumables with restrictions, preservatives, and extended shelf-life labels.

With its pesticides and herbicides, the agricultural industry bases some of its practices on the erroneous idea that plants share communicable diseases. But in fact, it's actually the soil's integrity and health that determine the wellness of the plants the industry grows. This is why sustainable/renewable farming should be the goal for all types of agriculture.

Since your interest in reading this book is learning how to use the terrain model to improve your own health, let's consider the hospital industry and all its different parts and departments. Of course, we want to go to clean hospitals, but these need not go overboard with bleach to kill off every tiny organism in them. Remember, precursors cannot be killed in the way we would recognize. Yes, bacteria can be killed off, at which point they return to their ancient dust forms.

Remember, bacteria are there only to help. Keeping things clean and fresh without chemicals is really all that is needed for us to reduce our exposure to toxins.

HMOs and the health-care insurance industry would not be able to sustain themselves if there were a decline in adherence to the germ theory because their practices and policies are designed for a system based on contagion. If a society knows that an illness is self-induced and people began taking responsibility for ensuring their symptoms are not being induced, then what would an HMO be needed for?

The ripple effect of believing in contagion is all too pervasive. If our society gave up the belief, we would even have to reevaluate our current educational materials containing historical references to contagious outbreaks that occurred throughout history in different cultures. Any industries and foundations that bank on the idea of finding a cure for disease would lose money and probably close shop.

If society recognized that our illnesses, diseases, syndromes, and infections are based upon our internal actions and how well we maintain our personal terrains, then all these industries would have to alter their activities to support society rather than taking advantage of it.

All the people employed by these industries would have to find new work, and the economy would undergo an upheaval while new businesses and industries and a new paradigm of thought were born based on a more accurate model that incorporates insights on the terrain.

It is each of our own responsibilities to recognize the choices we make and what impact they have on us and the world around us. Once a person comes to the conclusion that each and every person is deserving of the best for their health and well-being, they begin to make different choices. When enough of us reach the same conclusion, our new-paradigm thinking will halt industrial destruction.

What Shedding Belief in the Germ Theory Looks Like

If anything, shedding belief in the germ theory would provide people, communities, and all of humanity a grand opportunity to be more attuned to the natural way in which the body works. The ignorance and disregard promulgated by the germ theory would fade away and be replaced with a more wholesome, respectful, and sustainable view of each and everyone's body and the web that interweaves us with the plants and animals of the world. Presumed diseases and infections would almost be wiped off the planet because people would be educated from birth not to ingest chemicals or use them in the environment around their bodies.

People everywhere would do their best to ensure they did not interact with any substances—any chemicals, any humanmade products or toxins—that could reduce their vitality and possibly harm them. Thus, the companies creating those things would fail. All companies that wanted to thrive would have to be on their best behavior when designing their products.

Most importantly, we would all see that health for ourselves, for our world, and for future generations is built on the choices we make, not on the germs we blame.

Transcending the germ theory as a society will put an end to the unnecessary and counterproductive fight we are waging against our microscopic allies. And it will finally empower our symbiosis with nature. Not only will this create massive social change, but it will also create conditions for a world where all living organisms can thrive within balanced ecosystems.

THIRTEEN

□□□□□□□□

YOU ARE THE INHERITOR OF YOUR ANCESTORS' MICROBIOMES AND TERRAIN

"We cannot cheat Nature, by any means whatsoever—not by Christian Science, electricity, blood washing, or any other therapeutic measure. We still have to comply with Nature's laws or take our spanking."

HENRY LINDLAHR, M.D.

Health is the sum of all the effort and choices we make, actively and passively, consciously and unconsciously. Many people imagine that the state of health they experience over their lifespan is a foregone conclusion. They think their DNA predetermines everything: If Dad had high blood pressure, then so will Junior. If Mom developed dementia by age eighty, then so will Little Suzie when she's old. But in fact, our lifestyle choices give us more control over our health than is commonly realized. Epigenetic research has proven that the way our genes express themselves can be modified completely. It may even be possible to eliminate a predisposition at a deep cellular level.[1]

We don't have to think of ourselves as "people with diseases." You are not someone who is inheriting cancer or live forever with hypothyroidism, because your grandmother supposedly had it. It is common in our society for poor health to become an identity.

The truth is that we are the gardeners of our bodies' terrains. We are also stewards of the environment around us. That potentially gives us a lot of control over the kind of health that we will experience as individuals.

Claiming ownership of our health, among other things, requires us to develop a fundamental understanding of the synergy of the human body with the microbes on, in, and around it and help them do their tasks so that these friendly lifeforms will continue to sustain us. Believing that germs are enemies harming us while ignoring the destruction being wrought on our bodies by other things, such as pollution of the air, water, and soil, and consumption of chemically exposed and "genetically modified" monocrops and livestock is ignorant and self-defeating. It is our responsibility both to avoid harm and to supply ourselves with the nurturing that promote wellness.

I encourage you to cultivate a positive, synergistic view of your health.

The Influence of Our Parents on Our Biology

If you could instantly get an infection, then the reverse would be true also: You could instantly become healthy. Unfortunately, both ideas are mistaken. Neither getting sick nor getting well are instantaneous occurrences.

When we are working to bring our terrain into balance, the improvement of our health is usually gradual. Just as we have to work at becoming unwell, when we make the decision to restore our health or to take it to the next level, we have to allow the body time to do its work of coming back to being healthy.

It is possible that you have inherited a health advantage or disadvantage due to your ancestry. If you were born to two parents who were hugely aware of their health and took measures to maintain the balance of their terrain (even if they did not use this exact term), you would have started your life carrying a minimally toxic burden in your body, along with learning better adaptive behaviors during childhood than many of your peers.

After your parents taught you good habits, if you continued these habits into your adulthood, then you may be in relatively good condition right now, assuming that you have not been exposed to an inordinate amount of pollution, or injected with toxic chemicals.

Because of your parentage, you will have less of a propensity to display symptoms of imbalance than people whose parents did not take as good care of themselves as yours—because you inherited a body that has better efficiency to expel material that is detrimental and because you were taught how to maintain optimal wellness. As a result, you do not have to work as hard to be healthy as most folks. You essentially have inherited a more balanced body and mind.

One of the most important things you will inherit is a set of precursors. Through the extensive research that Dr. Enderlein did, he recognized that the sperm and the egg carried with it the precursors, which as you may recall he called *endobionts* (a combination of the words *endogenous* and *symbiotic).* The precursors, as you also learned earlier, maintain the cells and the terrain of the body. When and how our individual precursors respond to changes is unique to each of us. You inherit a unique combination of them from your parents, which means they adapt and respond to your terrain and environment uniquely for you.

Given that this is part of how parents give their offspring advantages and disadvantages, if you plan to become a parent, please understand that maintaining your internal health and the health of your partner will be essential for your child and future generations that arise from your union.

The beauty of taking care of your health is that when you have children of your own, after having done your best at maintaining your health, and especially if you are pro-creating with someone who has done the same, then your children will have even less of a hard time maintaining their good health than you do. You will contribute positively to their terrain and to their adaptability.

The responsibility of each individual descendent in a healthy sequence is only to continue to live as closely to nature's law—meaning to eat nutritious, nontoxic foods, wear natural fibers, and live in environments that place less stress on the body and mind. It is also to be connected with nature. The ease with which we should be able to live is similar to the ease of the people Dr. Weston A. Price studied in simple, preindustrial cultures in the early twentieth century.[2]

The harmonious nature with which we live in our surroundings and the positive influences of our parents and our community can promote balance within our bodies. Each of us is, by all rights, the microcosmic summation of our external societal and biological macrocosm, the precursors being the real cosmic primordial organisms that link it all.

Mentally, we may be living under stress because of fearing an invasion by microorganisms, because we have been indoctrinated with misguided notions about how our bodies maintain our wellness. Our skin, for example, is not the impenetrable fortress we may have been led to believe but a semipermeable covering that offers us an energetic as well as a physical exchange with the outside world. And the microbes that live on it are not our enemies, as our parents may have thought and taught us, but inherited friends, who are working relentlessly to help us continue making our personal journeys through life, translating both the energetic and physical stimuli of the external environment into a "language" that our nervous systems and inner worlds can comprehend and respond appropriately to.

Within all of us are seeds that were planted by our ancestors. The "seeds" are the information in our cells and precursors we inherit from them through the process of conception that occurs whenever a sperm enters an egg. Our embryonic cells carry the history of all of our ancestors' health that is our heritage. Cultures have referred to such particles as *ancestral dust*. This dust is the essence within us and around us of precursors that spring into action, supporting the life of your body.

You Are Not Your Symptoms

In current thinking, many of us identify ourselves by our symptoms and, especially, by medical diagnoses we receive. Unfortunately, because most of us live in a state of inadequate health, we have turned into a complacent culture that rewards disease and chronic illness with congratulatory accolades for surviving. This is not the way we should motivate ourselves to become optimally healthy. It is also not how we should teach future generations to live. Basically, we're just acquiescing to the prescriptions of a fundamentally flawed diagnostic health-care system.

Symptoms do not have to last forever. They are merely the way our bodies communicate what is happening to them and ask for attention. How our bodies communicate is similar to the way an infant cries for our attention: Words are not used. Rather, the guttural sounds the infant makes and its body language are how it tells us something isn't right. The body communicates through symptoms, such as sensations and color changes. Although we may not fully understand the language of the body, our job is to respond to these signs we perceive and make appropriate adjustments.

When we are feeling unwell, we should not identify with the symptoms our bodies are expressing. If anything, we should identify with the efforts and experiences that we utilize to create our health and well-being. The more we listen and respond to the voices of our precursors, inside and outside of our bodies, which at their root essence come to us from ancestors who lived in a very different, probably much cleaner environment than ours many generations ago, then it will be easier to attune ourselves to a more harmonious and balanced nature.

All of our thoughts, behavior, and actions either support or disrupt the balance in our bodies that these precursors—our ancestral dust—work hard to maintain. As an example, when we constantly react to situations with fear and anxiety, and harbor within us the thoughts of anticipating those situations, our imaginings create a reality for our brain and body. All parts of us spring into action, responding as if the thoughts are real. If this continues to happen, symptoms of imbalance start to display themselves from persistent wear-and-tear.

Ideally, when our health beliefs align with recognition of the sanctity of our bodies and utilize the knowledge from this book to help maintain our bodies symbiotically, we can reap the reward of the amazing benefits of clear thinking and vitality. We are the keepers of balance and guardians of health for our world and its future.

Like It or Not, Your Health Is Your Responsibility

Do you know why people believe the germ theory despite so much evidence disproving it? Because they prefer saying, "It's not my fault, it just happened." The germ-theory mentality allows people to avoid taking responsibility for anything that is happening to them or to their children. There's a comfortable simplicity in believing that one type of microorganism is responsible for an ailment, as it means there might be a single solution as well. Fix the one problem and—*voila!* —problem solved. People want to wrap their imbalances into nice, neat little packages of diagnoses, yet none of these artificial labels offers insight to the truth of the matter.

By contrast, the terrain paradigm mandates we take responsibility for ourselves. You cannot brush off signs of an imbalance and say that something outside you is at fault if you experience symptoms. Pus pouring out of a wound is not a sign of infection. It is a natural process in your body that helps it release a buildup of stuff it does not want in it and cannot tolerate anymore.

The terrain paradigm does not feed the childlike mentality of irresponsibility. It accepts that there are consequences to actions and behavior that don't reinforce or create a foundation for optimal health.

In our society, it's been rationalized all too often that we must continue to allow big businesses to market overconsuming, wasteful behavior to us. Proponents of germ theory embrace the mentality that products containing chemical ingredients (including known carcinogens that are deleterious to the body and environment), do not cause illness. But obviously, this is not true. Chemicals are toxic and can accumulate in our bodies, especially when there is imbalance. Repeated use of products containing harmful ingredients eventually will create changes on a deep, cellular level, if the body is unable to release them. This means they will be seen in both you and in your future offspring. But whether or not you decide to procreate, concern for our own well-being ought to last for the duration of our lives.

It is time for us to create a new view of health as a byproduct of personal responsibility, support of our natural physiological processes, and an emphasis on maintaining balance.

In his medical treatise *Airs, Waters, and Places*, written circa 400 BCE, ancient Greek physician Hippocrates writes: "Our natures are the physicians of our diseases."[3] He believed, as I do, that we have the natural ability to heal ourselves. This has always been true, yet the import of these words has not been truly heeded in the last hundred years or so. The symptoms of physiological imbalance in the body that modern medicine perceives as diseases are simply our bodies expressing their innate capacity for healing. They are attempting to correct an imbalance.

In other words, the symptoms *are* the remedy.

Techniques You Can Use to Support the Microbes Living in Your Body

What do we know about supporting our *microbiota* these days? The *micro* ("small") *biota* ("living things") inside our guts and on our skin. The microorganisms that live within us, on us, and around us, are essentially our precursors living in various locations in the terrains of our bodies, adapted to forms that are tasked to doing specific jobs in support of the respective locations they are found.

As you have learned, the precursors maintain the integrity of cellular function and communication along with making sure the function of excretion by cells and organs are maintained as well. When the terrain changes, they respond, pleomorphing into forms suited to the task of remediating the conditions in the surrounding ecosystem so it returns to optimal homeostasis.

The body's ecosystem is maintained by a series of complex interactions between various biological systems and the precursors in the forms of the microorganisms that coexist within it. This ecosystem is comprised not only of trillions of human cells but also of trillions of bacteria, mycobacteria, and so on—representing various pleomorphic forms that precursors take—working together. These microorganisms play a crucial role in maintaining homeostasis, aiding digestion, and supporting the regulation of the body by breaking down food, synthesizing essential nutrients from it, excreting waste products, and protecting against harmful toxins.

As I've referenced before, our whole body is essentially a garden. Now imagine that within this grand garden you also have smaller plots of land that host specific niche gardens. Every gardener would tell you that there are certain plants you don't grow with others, that there are certain plants that need specific soil or specific watering requirements. Each plant zone would then host different microorganisms, or even organisms that support it in its existence. Mutualism with cohabitation is a constant in the natural world, and this is where we can acknowledge that *is* what happens in our own bodies. For example, the nutritive and physiological requirements of your teeth are going to be different then the requirements of your eyeballs. Due to the abrasive nature of food consumption in the mouth, specific microorganisms are needed there which will help rehabilitate and repair gum tissue and the enamel of the tooth. Whereas in the terrain of your eyeballs, there's a form of lubrication and a protective coating and being that the eyeballs are utilized in a different way, and are fundamentally a completely different tissue, you will see different microorganisms in that location.

Seeing unfamiliar microorganisms, or a presence of them that is considered *pathological* by conventional science, gives us an understanding that some sort of deleterious exposure or disrupted cellular function has given rise to some sort of destruction. Following this observation, our job is to support the terrain by consuming the right nutrients, removing toxins, dealing with repair of the damage from the traumatic event. This is how we support our microscopic friends.

We can add more friends that help with various tasks in our body by consuming foods or taking specific remedies, like probiotic supplements, that resupply us.

The main task that we have to perform in order to maintain and restore the harmony of our inner universe is to pay attention to the needs and balance of the various micro terrains in our bodies. There are several ways we can do so, which I shall examine with you one by one—in no particular order of importance.

Probiotic supplementation. Much attention has been paid as of late to the benefits of dietary supplementation with probiotics. You've seen them mentioned on the labels of yogurt and kefir sold in your local grocery store as L. bacillus or L. thermophilus, and so forth. You've also seen them sold separately in powders that can be dissolved in water or juice or in capsules, by companies bragging how many billions are present. Probiotics are big business nowadays. Another form of probiotics are *isopathic remedies* that, unlike the classic form of probiotics, are the precursors in specific states of repair. These type of remedies can truly help support and enhance efficiency of your system's regulation, the way your body wants.

The primary question in regard to classic probiotics is, do we need to resupply our body's microbiome with additional precursors that have already assumed a bacterial form? And what can you expect when allowing your body's intelligence to provide its own natural healing responses with the support of the friendly microbiota you already possess? Consuming our foods unadulterated by industry and teeming with vitality (rich in precursors)provides a respect and understanding for our bodies, and we can live synergistically with the universe that is the body.

Eating vital, nutrient-dense foods. The best foods to consume are the ones our ancestors ate. They ate foods filled with vitality and nourishment along with minimal amounts of chemical contamination. As we supply ourselves with clean food, fresh air, and clean fresh water, we are resupplying ourselves with precursors already in a state of maintenance and communication.

Limiting or even more effectively removing industrialized processed foods that do not contain a richness of nutrients and the vibrancy of fresh, organic foods, helps reduce the strain that fake foods put on the body. The more you eat that doesn't supply you to refill your resources, the more deficient you will become and the more likely to experience toxic build up and imbalance.

Choosing the right food includes making sure that your proteins are sourced from animals and plants that have been treated well whose health was maintained throughout their lives. Just as our terrain changes because of toxins, malnutrition, and trauma, the terrain of animals and plants changes from exposure. The last thing that you would want to consume are foods that are mishandled and poorly treated, degenerated, and rapidly decomposing despite them looking not so bad.

The quality of the food you consume translates into the quality of the precursors you are taking into your own body. An example of this is when food is tested and found to have an excessive amount of unwanted bacteria. Obviously bacteria will be found in plants and animals that have died; but if a certain animal or plant has been contaminated by chemicals or was severely undernourished then the amount of decomposition because of excessive precursors pleomorphing into bacteria would be quite high.

Modern science misdirects our concerns toward the bacteria, when in fact we should be looking to the condition of the actual product. Its quality or lack of quality are a reflection of the conditions of its life.

Eating fermented foods. Not all decomposition is detrimental for human consumption. In fact, traditional fermented foods, such as yogurt, kefir, sauerkraut, kimchi, miso, kiviak, poi, and sourdough, among many others, provide an amazing assortment of nutrients and enzymes made by microorganic decomposition that will help enhance our digestion. These fermented foods contain a grandiose array of precursors that are working on breaking down material that actually did live a good, healthy life. In some cases, fermentation breaks down food components that otherwise would be inaccessible to us. Making it possible for humans to absorb nutrients makes these substances bioavailable and useful.

Another thing that many of the naturally fermented foods do which is of extreme importance is to help facilitate removal of harmful materials and excessive materials from the digestive tract when the body is having a hard time dealing with them on its own. You might say that fermented foods are facilitators of excretion.

When searching for fermented foods, it is important to note that some companies, including small businesses and farms, may use chemicals and stimulants in the production of fermented products which prevent natural fermentation from occurring. Natural fermentation is better.

Spending time in untouched natural landscapes. Being that the precursors are all around us, by spending time in natural environments that are untouched by human construction, like forests, jungles, and mountain areas, and even certain beaches and coasts, you can effectively saturate your body with more of the precursors. It is healthy to interact with pure, natural environments.

It's also important to be outdoors and get plenty of sunlight, as sunlight stimulates many of the processes within our body along with the precursors, plenty of fresh, clean water especially from untouched sources, and fresh air, which can be stimulating for the lungs and the sinuses.

Physical activity in natural environments has actually been shown, by conventional science, to positively influence the body's microbiota diversity.[4]

Reduce stress. Adequate sleep and management of stress, basically feed the part of the nervous system (the parasympathetic nervous system) that relaxes us, helps us digest, and enables us stay calm. Ensuring that there's balance within our nervous system, as well as that we get good nourishment and support, ensures proper communication between all systems within the body, including between the flora of the various microniches it hosts.

Calmness, serenity, mindfulness, and deep, healthy sleep keep the flow of blood to all the body in an even amount.

Balance in the nervous system reduces stagnation, over-utilization of resources, and proper adaptation to new stressors and outside environmental changes, including exposure to air pollutants and harmful electromagnetic frequencies. Making sure that your thoughts, habits, and activities bolster positive effects within your mind and your well-fed body.

It is important to know that the precursors and the microflora that they become will reflect the synergy and even flow of energy, blood, lymph, and nourishment throughout the entire body. Conducting ourselves with the understanding that our actions have an effect not only on our terrain but on the behavior of our precursors and the development of them into the optimal microbiome, will lead us to not suffer some of the most disabling symptoms of poor elimination. We must cooperate with the very actions our precursors take as they adapt to the ever changing landscape and are needed for digestion, assimilation, and elimination. Our cooperation with the precursor's integral role is essential for the body's systems integrity and efficient function. This mutualistic interdependence may be the most important factor in how healthy we can be. We are complex organisms, and we must not forget that our health is dependent on the way we treat our precursors.

Setting the idea of inheriting precursors aside, in all reality you control the shape of the precursors in your body—meaning you control how and when they pleomorph into saprophytes—through your decisions of what to eat and drink and how well you regulate factors in your life like stress. Thus, you are the architect of how your body expresses illness.

If you do not feed your terrain correctly, the choices you make will alter how the protectors of your blood, aka your precursors, take shape. Will they remain dormant or become microbes like bacteria, fungi, and helminths? You are in control of their metamorphosis, in control of how they react to their environment by what you feed them.

You control whether they pleomorph into a cleanup crew for your body or shift back into a less identifiable form that simply maintains and protects your cells.

Listen, Do Not Judge, and Participate

As the wise chiropractor William Trebing, D.C., states in his book, *Goodbye Germ Theory:*

> [Terrain] *theory laid out for us by Béchamp holds tremendous potential for the well-being of our planet here and now. It shows us that if we are responsible for our lives, if we manage our diets in a healthy fashion which is consistent with our species; if we maintain our fluid balance properly to persistently cleanse our circulatory and lymphatic systems; if we take more action to think and emote more positively, productively, and responsibly . . . clearly, the problem is not the microbe(s). The problem is the individual lifestyle which creates an*

environmental need for the production of virions, bacteria, and fungus.[5]

Signs from the body that reach the surface level are projections of deeper imbalances, and demonstrate that the body is slowly trying to correct many things; it just needs you to participate in helping it restore balance.

Our society imagines there is a black-and-white relationship of causality between specific microbes and specific diseases. Our belief in good and bad micro-organisms has led us to use a binary calculation to assess the value of a microbe's existence, and to take drastic measures to try to limit or destroy them in all avenues of life, creating imbalances in our bodies and disrupting our ecosystem.

At the time of this writing, for example, millions of chickens are being culled due to the belief that a virulent microorganism (avian influenza) may cause illness in both chickens and those who consume them. But look at the crowded and dirty conditions in which many chickens are being raised, the quality of their feed, and the antibiotics with which they are dosed. If the chickens are sick, it should call into question the methods of animal husbandry used to keep them alive and fatten them up for human consumption. It is a clue for us that something in the operation of these industrial farms has gone wrong. Both their environment and their food supply must be toxic. The microorganisms in the chickens' bodies are engaged in bioremediation of these animal and their environments.

The idea that there are good germs and bad germs, even within the context of an altered, degraded terrain, exists nowhere else in nature other than in our minds and literature. Nature sees neither good nor bad, only function and balance.

For example, a lion is not seen as bad because it eats an antelope; this is just how it is. Predators play a role in maintaining the natural balance of their ecosystem. They ensure a niche is not overrun by prey animals to the point of overconsumption and trampling of plants. Predatory animals also ensure the survival of the most fit prey animals, which pass their strengths on to their offspring.

For their part, antelopes and other prey animals ensure that predators are limited in their numbers, by maintaining robust vitality within the herd. In doing so, they limit access to their culling since they would be harder to catch.

Back to our germs. Because we are looking at them outside the context within which microorganisms function, it is us who have assigned the morality of good and evil to the natural functions of microorganisms. Removing these organisms from the environment they inhabit, or simply changing the environment, and they cease to function, or even to exist in their known form altogether. This is why our lifestyle choices, have the most significant impact on our well-being.

Your Terrain Is the Sum of Your Choices

The whole point of the terrain paradigm is empowerment of the individual. All of this is to understand that what we call symptoms of *illness* are not random. Good health or poor health is a consequence of the choices we make. It is not brought about either by misfortune or through the opportunism of microscopic particles floating in the air.

FOURTEEN

□□□□□□□□

BREAK THE SPELL OF GERM THEORY EVERYWHERE

"Germs do not cause any disease. . . . There is more harm in the fear of germs than there is in the germs themselves."

SIMON LOUIS KATZOFF, M.D.

Now that you know microorganisms do not cause diseases but are actually helping us restore our bodies to the state of optimal health, it is going to begin to dawn on you how much wasted effort and money in our lives and society can be attributed to blind reliance on the polarizing belief in the germ theory. That recognition may make you sad. It could enrage or frustrate you. But in the end, it is liberating to become aware that you cannot randomly "catch" a microbe. You get to reclaim your time, energy, and mental focus, and make different and better choices.

The effort you put into the well-being of your physical body and your mind from now on, based on your new understanding of how optimal health comes about, will eventually be fruitful. Nothing really can diminish all the efforts you make to support your body and mind, improve the condition of the environment around you.

I suspect you've been reading this book because you're eager to be free of the control of corporations that profit off people's poor health and free of fear from nonexistent dangers exposed by supposed health experts all the while dismissing the importance of your own symbiosis. And reading also because you want to live and/or raise your kids in a healthful environment and leave the world in a better place than you found it. If you are like the people who come to me for advice in my terrain-model wellness practice, then you mainly want to live in peace and harmony as naturally as possible.

The germ theory is a subversive lie. It has given people the idea that we can be *invaded* or *assaulted* by nature surreptitiously, and that no matter what we do, there will always be something lurking around us that can override all the good work we put into being healthy. The insidious concepts of *contagion* and *infection* make us believe that we can host a party of uninvited guests inside our bodies. But in fact, the "party" in the body is of our own making.

Everything that is happening to your body and the bodies of your family members, including the nourishment they receive and the toxins you choose to allow to be present in the environment around you, is based on the success of your efforts of keeping a balanced terrain, inside and out, and your willingness to learn. The joint efforts of every individual in a community making and adhering to healthful, life-sustaining policies matter, too.

On a corporate-influenced, political level, the germ theory has influenced the marketplace for decades by disrupting the natural choices people make for the benefit of themselves and their community. For instance, instead of supporting local, chemical-free farming practices, many people are bamboozled into buying cheaper produce that must be transported to them from farther distances. These most likely were sprayed with pesticides.

Another example is how many people do not question the contamination of municipal water systems that have chemicals put in them to "kill germs," although the use of many of those additives is supported by limited scientific safety and efficacy studies. These mistakes cripple the natural development of healthy, self-sustaining systems in our communities. We are living with, and future generations will be growing up with, an unfortunate dependency on corporate-created products and services that cause harm. Our rampant consumerism, which is underpinned by obfuscated corporate agendas, extends into the realm of environmental regeneration and sustainability—and health advocacy, too. Mislabeling of products, for example, with marketing terms like *green* and *natural* is just another way that corporations take advantage of us.

There are social justice issues at stake in balancing the terrain of our society. People in low-income neighborhoods often find themselves residing in so-called *green deserts* without access to street trees, parks, gardens, surrounded by cell phone towers, electric lines, and vehicle exhaust. Industrial plants that spew chemical waste into air and water are located near them.

It is beholden on all of us to ensure corrective measures are taken. We cannot strive to be optimally healthy unless everyone and everything is considered relevant to the process. The wave of advocacy and environmental measures our society is in the midst of taking now reflects the reality of what's actually good for business. What's best is the opposite of polluting the world to make a buck. As the environmentalist and U.S. Secretary of Health and Human Services Robert F. Kennedy, Jr., has said: "Good environmental policy is good economic policy."[1]

The celebrated social activist Mahatma Gandhi taught us to be the change we want to see in the world. The reason that this principle is so empowering to embrace is that it stops us from acting like victims and invites us to become leaders. Gandhi's beliefs help convey the importance of choice on our own lives as well as on the community. As an example, Gandhi understood the impact of fasting as an act of purification for his body (microcosm) and its impact on British negotiations (macrocosm). His choices, just as our choices, impact society and the landscape around us. The choice to fear the idea of contagion reflects the absence of a community ethos in many industrialized nations. It represents our lack of an overt trust and symbiosis with nature and to one another.

The uncertainty that germ theory has created in humanity—collectively—has caused many of us to seek solace and comfort in health-care solutions and products supplied by companies like those in the pharmaceutical industry, which are run by profiteers who bank on their ability to hire cheap labor and sell consumers medicines that are unneeded.

When symptoms of detoxification are misconstrued by doctors and researchers as negative phenomena, companies respond by creating antibiotic, antiparasitic, symptom-suppressive medications and inoculations.

The notions of disease as random occurrences or condemning acts of God, or worse, as the result of curses from demonic forces, can be dissolved by learning that symptoms are not random, but also not bad things either. Symptoms really are something to be understood and embraced.

Every choice you make will impact you, whether or not the impact is beneficial. The benefit depends on how the choice is handled inside your body. Take empowerment from knowing you can choose your path of adding to or detracting from your health.

Embrace the Magic

The body is a strong organism, almost to its own detriment, because of being able to host so many noxious substances. Despite being in almost complete imbalance at times, still it survives! The body can withstand tremendous abuse, withstanding horrid situations, such as malnutrition, dehydration, exposure to radiation and pollution, violence, and emotional pressure, and it survives.

The body is magical. Made from the dust of our ancestors and particles of our planet carried on the winds of time, it is our legacy as children of the Earth. Germ theory denies the magic of the body's symbiosis with the microbes in, on, and around it, and, in the place of magic, generates fear of the very beings that help us continue living and eventually to thrive.

If we could randomly get sick, what would be the point of natural medicine—herbology, homeopathy, acupuncture, naturopathy, and more? Germ theory does not provide hope. The terrain model *does*. And beyond hope, this model gives us the understanding to know that we can always become experientially better, stronger, and wiser from the negative forces our bodies endure by many of these toxic exposures, just as a sapling growing in a forest does from the onslaught of weather changes.

One important aspect of the terrain paradigm is becoming genuinely aware of and connected to your body and mind. Start paying attention to all the processes that are occurring. What are you thinking? What are you feeling? Do you feel physically and mentally in balance? This will help you avoid falling prey to health schemes that do nothing more than line the pockets of shareholders.

People need to be "sick" for drug makers to profit. If you are balanced and optimally healthy, maintaining your health should not be a source of cash for profit-driven corporations.

History and current events have shown us that fear rules the thinking in many scientific fields of study. If fear rules the thinking of scientists, then experiments in different fields may be done in error by them. Countless times, scientists of antiquity were commissioned to quell the fires of fear with supposed scientific provings that supported opportunistic capitalism, either made in haste or completely fabricated, in order to support the gains of a rich few. The germ theory was one of those fabrications, though not the only one that the health industry is driven by.

And the fact is that our entire modern medical system is today reliant on this ideology for diagnoses and treatments, yet it continues to fall short of curing millions of people of their simple ailments daily. This is evidence that the system is failing miserably. Too many people are even going bankrupt in an attempt to cover the cost of medical bills that pay for treatments which do not work as intended.

We submit to embracing the germ theory at our own peril.

The inconsistency of the contagious-microbe model persists, yet the propagated fear within most of humanity remains. Germ theory is fear based.

Naturopathic doctor William Freeman Havard, N.D., in the early twentieth century, said:

> *Fear and impatience are two factors which tend to delay complete recovery. Fear lowers the vitality, and impatience leads to the dangerous practice of aborting or suppressing the reaction. If the patient's mind can be released from the grip of fear, whether it be a concrete fear of impending death or the vaguer fears generated in him by his helplessness, the battle is half won.*[2]

Naturopathic doctor Louis Kuhne, N.D., said:

> *All the various forms of disease are, as we have seen, only efforts of the body to recover health.*[3]

We have nothing to fear from our body's cries for help in supporting it. It is this mindset that holds us back from reaching the ultimate goal of real health.

New Terminology Leads to Better Thinking

Even if you fear the idea of exposure to a supposed germ, it doesn't change the fact that you cannot "catch" anything. Your fear of being infected by a microscopic organism is a fiction propagated by advertisers efforts at controlling your ability to think for yourself. They deliberately reinforce the disempowering belief that your health is out of your control. This terminology of *catch* or *infect* is a constant, highly prevalent splinter in the skin of humanity. We see these words in everything, not just health. The repetition of these words, along with the mindset of what these words mean, fortifies the "catching" standard of thinking in the subconscious.

To create a new mindset, we have to understand that not only must we change the words we use to describe our healing processes and functions, but we must also alter our perception of the events which we refer to as *illness*.

If someone says, "I am sick," we have to look for what is really happening. Are they displaying symptoms of an internal event? No matter the symptoms, whether as simple as sneezing and coughing or as severe as fevers, rashes, and vomiting, all are signs of the removal of toxins and decomposition and of the rebalancing being undergone to re-establish homeostasis.

Many practitioners who are like-minded to me will utilize words that emphasize the importance of recognizing the body's signs. Words and phrases that have been used instead of *catching a cold* or *getting sick* are:

- *Detox.*
- *Upgrade.*
- *Download.*
- *Transform.*
- *Transmute.*
- *Shift.*
- *Let go.*
- *Release.*
- *Recharge.*
- *Purge.*
- *Flush.*
- *Cleanse.*

And so many more.

These terms can help us step away from the misguided idea of germ transference. Making use of them helps us understand that we can catch the wave of detoxing, balancing, or upgrading our biological systems to support a better and more efficient internal ecosystem in accordance with the ever changing landscape of our external.

We have to fully appreciate and become wholly aware that we are social creatures. There will always be an exchange or communication beyond our true comprehension, like all animals, plants, and other organisms that socialize.

Let us not get distracted by the negative insinuations and logical fallacies of stifled scientists who still, to this day, do not understand why we yawn when someone else does. Instead let's make a new way of thinking contagious—our understanding regarding our health using these words.

The word *prevention* is, most importantly, a word we need to adjust in our health terminology. Using the word *prevention*, we may imagine that our whole lives are just holding back an inevitable affliction we assume we will one day have. It's as if we are holding back a tsunami of disease.

What kind of mindset is that? To call naturopathic, chiropractic, or even nutrition "preventative" is to completely disregard what people practicing these disciplines are actually doing. Naturopathy, for instance, is a teaching of sustainability by supporting the body to the fullest.

Recalling the concept of your body as a garden landscape—your inner terrain—may help you to flip to this alternate way of thinking. With what kind of mentality do you want to define your existence? Living in the mentality of prevention means believing that factors that keep you from being optimally well, no matter how big or small they are, are outside your control and therefore threatening. It's as if you live in a castle and must build and maintain a fort around it to protect yourself against the evil designs of a warlord wanting to come in and take over.

Consuming foods that are fresh and clean—and appropriate for your body—can correct structural imbalances and encourage the flow of blood and lymph in your body. This is not *preventative* care, it's health *maintenance.* It's not fort building, which is preventative in nature; it's building and maintaining a network of communication and friendly collaboration within the body and outside in the community.

Good self-care maintains and improves our bodily systems so that they function at their most optimal level every day. The mentality of maintenance is glass-*full* (as opposed to *half-full)* thinking. The intent is to create resources and resilience. And it becomes easier as you build on it, day after day.

The idea of prevention in the germ theory world is a corruption of this approach. The idea of prevention is glass-half-empty thinking. It is based on the notion that something dangerous is inevitably around the corner, waiting to make you sick. The way we are taught prevention in our society gives us the impression that sometimes, no matter how great an effort we make to build an impenetrable castle around us, something will always eventually get through our defenses. Any time prevention is presented as a metaphorical fort holding germs, diseases, and death at bay, it makes us afraid.

This is not so. In the terrain model, the actual model of health, the model that nature and all of the animal, plant, microbiological worlds within it follow, exemplifies the premise that positively building the body—for example, by limiting toxins, eating well, and taking other actions—reduces the likelihood of buildup and degeneration of tissues. The more you build, the better you feel. You are building a bank account of good health. The more "capital" you put into it, the more "interest" it earns. In this case, the interest comes in the benefits of vibrancy, vitality, and optimal excretion of noxious substances.

Nothing is attacking. Nothing is random. Nothing can be attributed to luck.

Another deleterious mindset is falling into the trap of thinking *It's genetic*. This idiom needs to be adjusted. Yes, a predisposition can be inherited—but in a way that means you have to work harder to strengthen your system as a whole. The need to make an effort does not absolve you of responsibility to maintain balance in your terrain. Avoid making the assumption that there's nothing you can do "because *it's genetic*."

Our familial and microbial inheritance from our parents is dynamic (just like the value of the funds in the bank accounts and stock portfolios we inherit) because it is ever influenced by our behaviors and environment.

Epigenetics is the study of how your behaviors and the environment can affect and alter the way your body expresses itself—altering the expression can be likened to flipping on-and-off switches. You can turn off a "switch" you inherited that was in an "on" position. And then potentially pass this beneficial expression on to your own babies.

Though this insight is more flexible, it still leaves little to the nuance of our existence. If we submit to thinking the expression of our innate tendencies cannot be changed, we allow the manifestations of trauma passed on to us to repeat until the body is exhausted into a chronic illness.

If you live your life fearing a possible disease phenomenon or contagion, you will have little time or, for that matter, limited rational thought with which to be able to do anything else with complete freedom. Fear itself can cause changes in our structure and healing capabilities and can alter our state of health. Scientist Masaru Emoto proved this in his experimentation with the impact of positive and negative messages on frozen water. He studied how the emotions of each type of word affected the way water crystallized. When a word taped to a water glass conveyed a universal positive emotion, the crystals made from the water were symmetrical and beautiful. When the words elicited a universal negative emotion, like hatred or anger, the crystals never really formed well.

Many if not most of what is considered holistic medicine and all sorts of well-meaning practitioners have succumbed to using concepts like *diagnosis*, *prevention*, *vulnerability*, and *genetic inheritance* as part of their process of healthcare. Holistic healthcare is fundamentally the belief of empowerment and understanding of the interaction of humanity and nature, which are great intentions and that is what needs to be focused on.

Yet how does prevention-type terminology bolster the self-confidence of a person seeking natural medicine? From my perspective, it doesn't. Insidiously, this terminology can subconsciously create doubts in people's minds that they are not doing enough to stave off disease.

Another fallacy propagated by many health-care practitioners is that a person will have a diagnosis or disease forever, meaning that they will need to take synthetic supplements, follow specialized diets, and received constant therapies for the rest of their lives to stave off the unfortunate inevitability of their condition. This just feeds into the victim mentality.

Change Your Words Because You Are Not a Victim

"Enlightenment is the unlearning of the thought system that dominates the planet."[4]

MARIANNE WILLIAMSON

Because of constant brainwashing from the perpetual reinforcement of the germ theory in our society, many people try to fit the idea of the terrain model into their preexisting germ/contagion paradigm of belief, knowingly or unknowingly integrating the two as one. Many integrative physicians and nutritional specialists, for example, will insert ideas of contagion into their discussions of the terrain model, either due to their lack of comprehension of pleomorphism or over reliance of the germ theory to diagnose their patients.

Health-care practitioners who are also entrepreneurs often reframe the terrain model for their own purposes, such as selling industrially made probiotic supplements or detoxification agents. Because they believe in contagion, they are eager to offer their customers and patients some sort of literal rescue device.

When the human body is engaged in purging toxins and repairing its cells and tissues, processes associated with detoxification, the body emits an energetic field that could impact other people who come into contact with it conceivably. But I prefer using the word *connection* to describe this phenomenon, rather than the word *contagion*—particularly when I am talking about health care in a group setting, since contagion is an involuntary communication that implies negativity.

The prevailing mindset of victimization is irksome to me because it negates the truth of our sovereignty over our bodies. It implies that we are acted upon by the world involuntarily. Whether conscious or unconscious of the exchanges we have with other people on the biological and energetic levels, I believe the words *connection* and *communication* connote that we are engaged in making a *voluntary* choice to exchange or connect with the world around us.

Contagiousness is the centerpiece of the germ theory model of health. One trouble I have with this model is that it does not amply recognize the impact of communication between intersecting energy fields, electrons, cells, humans, animals, the precursors, and so on. The exchanges between organisms may one day be established to be on a measurable level for current science and must be incorporated in our view of healthy environment.

So, from now on, *contagious* is not the word to be used if we believe in the terrain model. Practitioners especially need to step away from utilizing words and patterns that promote the idea of contagious germs. The germ theory fundamentally promotes and reinforces that all processes in our bodies are involuntarily happening, while many processes are based on fortune and luck. This is not science or truth. Yogis, hypnotists, and behavioral scientists have shown time and time again that our minds, either consciously or subconsciously, can manipulate and even control almost every bodily function, including our perception of pain.[5]

By removing terminology that promotes belief in *infections* or *catching* germs, we reduce our fear of vulnerability or being weak. In essence, we cannot reinforce our lack of vulnerability to catching something that cannot be caught. Logically, in any regard, we cannot be vulnerable to a contagion.

Making this change removes the overused word *fight* from the context of health care. If the saprophytes (bacteria and such) are helping us, we really are NOT fighting them. As there is no need to resist a natural detoxification process, our bodies are never *fighting a cold*, for instance. Or *battling* cancer.

All the germ theory does is promote words that insinuate we are engaged in a violent, ongoing struggle with nature, a negative emphasis that creates an embattled mentality. We are not at war with our precursors. Nor do we need to war with or fear each other's presence. Nobody is a "carrier" of germs because nefarious germs don't exist.

Also, we are not at war with ourselves and our bodies. We live in a dynamic of balance and harmony and have to embrace all functions of the body, whether they connote a condition of harmony restored or a state in which we are currently detoxing.

Everything We Need Is Inside Us

We must set aside egotistical, reductionistic views of the body if we want to integrate the belief that each body is a natural, symbiotic, synergistic, and dynamic organism which has its own individual expression of health—an expression that fluctuates based on both internal and external factors.

Observations of culture, gender, stress, environment, toxic exposure, and any other variations should be considered when we seek to build a particular body's resources. Naturopathic practitioners can help you measure the impact of such factors on your physical, mental, and emotional state of being. The measurement of toxic stressors can help to elucidate and clarify any connection that exists to a multitude of symptoms your body is displaying.

If we look at other mammals living in a variety of environments, some more hostile than our own, we can see that they adapt rather quickly to changes by mentally and physically accepting the changing, allowing the body to produce all sorts of enzymes and antitoxins. Interestingly enough, the simple creation of antitoxins for tetanus and diphtheria are manufactured by this method, but in an artificial way in a laboratory. Scientists inject a toxin into an animal, then withdraw its blood after it has adapted. The mammal's body creates the antitoxin that members of our species use to (supposedly) prevent disease.

Now, if another type of mammal can produce an antitoxin, who is to say human beings could not produce similar antitoxins ourselves? Is science giving the healthy human body a chance to develop antitoxins? Or is it that we cannot actually find a healthy human whose body can produce the antitoxin we are looking for? Do we have the correct tools to measure the nuances of adaptation? Do we know what we are looking for in the first place or is current science a horse with blinders?

Have scientists really taken the time to study the human body's full capabilities, or have they closed the book on further investigation since they believe that "preventative" vaccines are the best solution anyone could ever find?

I refer you now to the example of certain snake masters who have either allowed venomous snakes in their care to bite them repeatedly or who have intentionally injected minute amounts of snake venom into themselves to deliberately prompt adaptation. These people's bodies, over time, possibly produce, for a lack of better words, natural antitoxins/antivenins. Thus, if they are bitten again by accident, little to no symptoms arise. They live even though another person bitten by the same snake might die of venom poisoning.

This is evidence that given enough time and support, the human body can create what it needs in order to balance itself out. Due to our individuality, not everyone will produce an antitoxin or adapt to eliminating the metabolites of the broken down toxin during the same time frame or in the same way. Each response from each of us is unique, yet, because we are all human, there will be always some similarity in the way our bodies respond to substances we encounter.

This is obviously an oversimplification of how our bodies work. Individual people inherit different propensities from their parents that allow them to adapt better or worse to certain environments, foods, and toxic substances. All of us would benefit from taking inventory of our own health standing, inheritances, and upbringings to really understand and appreciate our personal capabilities.

Most importantly, what actually needs to be done when we're ailing, on many occasions, is to rest for the sake of recuperation. Rest, along with other supportive therapies, gives the body a chance to cope with the stressors affecting it. Convalescence is how we make time and give support to the body.

This advice is not taught or reinforced by the conventional medical model, and frankly, it is infrequently taught and reinforced in the holistic world as well. Our impatience with recuperation and demand for quick fixes has backed us into a corner of relying on a model of false diagnoses and synthetic, victim-based cures.

Aim to appreciate the strong desire of your body to be in balance, physically and energetically, and cultivate faith in the idea that it has the faculties to do so. With knowledge and recognition of the holism of body, mind, and spirit, and how we all contain unfathomable abilities to restore our natural harmony when it has been pushed out of balance, we should begin to create a new model of health. A new terrain medicine.

AFTERWORD

□□□□□□□□□

EVOLVE YOUR HEALTH-CARE OPTIONS

Working off of the understanding that there is no such thing as a virus or an ability to spread a contagion manufactured in a laboratory, I propose that we evolve both our view of how to make ourselves healthier and our health-care options. The principles of terrain medicine could guide us to devise new public health policies (as well as stricter environmental policies) going forward that are more effective, less toxic, and less expensive.

If we were to drop the cognitive influence of the germ theory, what would be an appropriate response when significant numbers of people simultaneously and suddenly get the same symptoms of disease in the future? How might we prepare for this as individuals? How might we prepare as a society? And who are the experts we should turn to in a crisis like the so-called COVID-19 pandemic?

To explain my thinking, I will share a few ideas I have about what started the pandemic in 2020 that led to lockdowns, mask-wearing, and horrid hospital policies for several years after. The year 2020 was a turbulent, mishandled year of exposure to toxins and poor health-care protocols. Many governments and companies utilized chemicals that caused the very symptoms their staff members blamed on a fictitious, never isolated virus. Between the exaggerated flu vaccine rollout, weather modification chemicals, and the toxic soup spewing forth from industrial plants, we witnessed weaponized toxicity on a massive scale.

Add to the fear created by the media, a political coverup similar to a coverup regarding the swine flu vaccine that occurred in 1976, evidence of countries abusing chemical sanitizers, and overconsumption of synthetic vitamins by the public, and we had ourselves a pseudo-pandemic. Severe, frequently fatal symptoms were experienced on a massive scale only within a hospital setting. One of the symptoms most noted was people's loss of their sense of smell. But the simple use of zinc in weather modification, metallurgy, hand sanitizers, and synthetic vitamin tablets could be one reason to explain this loss.

My advice for avoiding a similar "outbreak" of disease in the future is to stop fearing fictional germs and start following the money trail until we can identify who profits from it. It is the profiteers, the people chasing profits from medications and therapies, who are largely responsible for destroying the environment of the Earth and making everybody sick.

In 1921, naturopath Benedict Lust wrote:

> [Man] *has surrounded himself with all manner of unnatural conditions, built himself an environment that*

> *reacts upon him every minute of his life, loads his digestive organs with the most ungodly foods, filling his body with poisons and when nature finally calls him to account he looks for a panacea that will relieve his suffering but at the same time permit him to continue with his acquired habits of life.*[1]

It is because of this mentality that people can be easily profited off of. Blaming a germ, of course, relieves a person of their responsibility for having an unhealthy lifestyle.

How can anyone say we know conclusively how any microorganism functions, especially when a health condition has arrived at the point of end-stage cellular deterioration? By then, the body is riddled with decay and all kinds of microbes that would not be present in the body of an optimally healthy person. Does the fact that particular bacteria exist in great quantities in the sick person's body indicate that they were a factor in the original development of the disease? Or could it actually be that the level of cellular death is so great that the body itself is creating the toxins in its own tissues that a conventional physician would attribute to disease-creating organisms that produce enterotoxins?

My professional opinion is that physical changes cause the body's state of sepsis.

Is it hard for you to believe that you cannot "catch" a cold—or any other disease? Think about why that may be the case. Does it make you feel better to believe that your cold is random or that the infection you're experiencing in your lungs is not your fault? Is taking responsibility for your ailments and imbalance something beyond your ability to comprehend? Or something that just sounds too difficult to do well?

The theory of health that is currently supported *en masse* by most health practitioners, conventional and holistic alike, is saturated with superstition, and all basic principles of science are violated at the very start. It is because of these false beliefs, these longstanding superstitions of contagion, that we give companies the opportunities to sell remedies and poisons to us that just make our bodies sicker. And though some people get temporary relief from these remedies, they know deep down that their imbalances, their "diseases," are becoming more serious.

Many people want to pinpoint specific culprits for their conditions, whether they are experiencing symptoms of lung cancer, ebola, or flu. My contention is that in every instance of poor health, a toxin is always present, either by exposure or by internal creation, causing our symptoms. If we were to isolate people showing limited to no effects of disease during any epidemic, we'd find that they have a strong underlying foundation of good health and excellent nutrition that is boosting their natural ability to detoxify and heal, all the while resonating vibrancy and resilience. What is key for them is the efficiency with which their bodies work.

Does modern science truly know what constitutes a healthy person? Does it know how someone like that stays healthy? Importantly, science at present has little to no clue on how to turn "sick" people into healthy ones.

Begin by Respecting Yourself as a "Whole" Being of Magnificence

Medicine and the field of conventional healthcare are filled with many well-intentioned people who are immersed in a paradigm of quick fixes and false statistics. Because conventional thinking is prevalent in our society, it is easy to become conditioned to believe that without antibiotics to kill bacteria and chemotherapy to kill tumor cells our bodies would succumb to degradation and death. More so, we have family and friends around us who, by expressing their fears to us, may pressure us to accept the paradigm and eventually sabotage any questioning of the medical system that we do. The first step in evolving your health-care options is to avoid getting lost in a tornado of fear, confusion, coercion, and lack of faith in your human body.

Remember these two things:

1. Your body knows best.
2. When you listen to, and act upon, your body's messages, you will know best what measures are appropriate for you to take.

Stop allowing profit-making companies, not to mention doctors and politicians, to dictate whether you have an illness, a contagious microbe, or the need for their products. Stop them from trying to control your decisions about how to care for the needs of your individual body.

In reality, as Melvin Page, D.D.S., and H. Leon Abrams, Jr., point out in their book *Your Body Is Your Best Doctor*: "Good health and cures are often brought about merely by correcting body chemistry. In this approach, the patient must be treated not just for the specific part of the body which noticeably ails him, but for his entire body since each minute part is merely an interacting part of the whole."[2]

The approach of detoxifying the body is appropriate for the treatment of all ailments and so-called infections. The body is one functioning whole, even though conventional medicine addresses deleterious reactions emerging from different body parts as separate issues. Each of us is a whole unique organism constantly responding to daily doses of inner and outer toxins.

Furthermore, understanding our uniqueness, as individuals with our own needs and unique requirements for health, should be the key element in a plan for bolstering our vitality and establishing optimal health. It is difficult to apply a specific protocol for the totality of humanity for a particular problem, even partially. Many factors need to be considered before a doctor can appropriately prescribe natural medicines and a diet for an individual. Factors such as ethnicity, behavioral heredity, current living status, working conditions, and even the age group of the individual have to be taken into account. Understanding that the microorganisms living synergistically within us and around us are highly influenced by the nourishment and treatment of the body tells us it is in our best interest to understand our own needs.

Page and Abrams assert: "A specific diet cannot be prescribed as being good for everyone in that each person has a distinct heredity and has varied experiences in his environment . . . A good diet is always beneficial to health, and a poor diet is always injurious to health. The degree to which a bad diet manifests itself depends upon the hereditary constitution of the person concerned."[3]

If a poor diet continues, then symptoms of disease will eventually manifest, indicating to the person who's been eating poorly that they need to change their ways. This is the time when it is extremely important for such a person to heed the warnings so they can avert their emerging symptoms before falling into a deeper hole of deficiency, inflammation, and pain. This is true even if the person thinks they are already following the "best" diet or a "healthy" diet.

The root of all disease stems from traumas impacting already imbalanced and severe, long-standing deficiencies that exist within the body's tissues and cells. Constant abuse impregnates this patterning deep within the system. You could say these are the root causes of all disease, even though people will usually display their imbalances and deficiencies in different ways. Imbalances can be present at birth, or they can slowly progress throughout our lives, due to our exposure to chemicals in our environment (even something as seemingly innocuous as a synthetic cleaning product), slowly and gradually manifesting into symptoms within the body. As more contaminants and malnourishment affect us, our bodies adapt to the new internal and external environment we're immersed in to stay alive.

This is a homeoregulatory, adaptive response.

Adaptation to our surroundings on the level of our cells is how our species evolves. The supposed epidemics and waves of illnesses sweeping through whole populations that we've seen in our historical records are examples of the human body's adaptive measures. These not only ensure a proper detox for each individual, but also enable people to "download" information about current changes in the environment (physical, energetic and otherwise) and how to handle and excrete whatever the negative stimuli in an environment may be so that young people who are procreating will pass this cellular information on to members of future generations. Their descendants will be ready to handle those same stimuli with little effort.

Louise Lust, N.D., a heroine of early naturopathic medicine, simply said, "If mothers would learn how . . . to prepare simple healthy food and by example teach their children the all-important lessons of how and what to feed their body, sickness would be outgrown and forgotten in one generation."[4] And I agree with her. We need to get back to the simplicity of understanding the human body as a whole organism, not just as a bunch of cells and systems. The body is a beautiful, harmonious universe, with parts that are dependent and independent at the same time.

Making our lives complex by exposing ourselves to constant emotional, physical, and spiritual crises without reprieve will eventually lead to a buildup of toxic material in our bodies and minds. But even when that happens, as chemist James C. Thomson, Sr., writes in his classic 1939 book *The Heart:* "I believe that Nature Cure people are right when they apply to physical disease the same method that we apply to psychical disease. Just as a buried wish should be lived out, so should a buried poison be allowed to find its way out," then our unrestricted and properly supported bodies will know what to do.[5]

Nature is wise in this manner.

ACKNOWLEDGMENTS

I'd like to take this opportunity to express my gratitude to the many people who influenced, helped, and supported me in the making of this book.

First and foremost, my husband, Louis Belchou, without whom none of this would be possible. Your countless hours of transcribing my gibberish, helping me connect the dots, researching by my side, enduring the towers of books and paperwork in every room, and doing countless chores will always be a reminder to me of your selflessness, support, confidence in me, and love.

My two beautiful and smart girls. I will be in your debt forever for giving me the space and time to write this book for you and the generations to come. Thank you, my darlings.

My sister, Michelle Arce. Thank you for keeping me well-nourished and entertained.

I am grateful to my mother, Janet Arce, who, since I could open my mouth and started to question what I was being taught, educated me and pushed me to speak up and tell the truth.

My editor, Stephanie Gunning. Words cannot convey how appreciative I am. Your faith in my writing skills still amazes me. Your egging me on provoked some of my best work. Thank you.

Melanie Ryan, you ignited the flame of writing in me when you insisted I take everything I know and put it on paper. Thank you. I would also like to thank Andy Steigmeier (and Justin, I know you are watching) for keeping me laughing. Sometimes the greatest ideas come when one is most at peace.

When I was jumping headfirst into the rabbit hole of information about the lies of the germ theory, I came across the work of Dr. Will Trebing. Thank you for your knowledge and book, *Goodbye Germ Theory*. It opened my eyes.

Thank you, Lisa Moore and Lisa Rooth, for your encouragement and gung-ho cheerleading. Your jovial support kept me lighthearted throughout the book writing process.

Thank you, Lara Tabaznik and John Tsafos, for your encouragement as I journeyed to publish this book. I am grateful to you for connecting me to people who would help ensure that these words would be seen by many.

Dr. Christiane Northrup, you are an inspiration to me, and a legend. Thank you for being a pioneer and advocate for true healthcare, and forging the road ahead for me.

Dawn Lester, thank you for taking the time to talk with me and looking over my work. Your proofreading is impeccable. The book that you and David Parker wrote, *What Really Makes You Ill?*, should be a staple in everyone's home as it is in mine.

I am grateful to all the wonderful clients and friends who have listened to the advice of this "crazy" doctor over the years. Your trust in my guidance has motivated me and spurred me on to teach others.

All the loving and beautiful animals and plants in my life, you have been my wisest teachers, showing me the truth about nature and true biology.

I wish to express my gratitude to Sally Fallon Morell and the Weston A Price Foundation for all the accrued sacred knowledge and amazing fortitude I have learned from you through the years. Your work has reinforced my core belief system that "health is wealth" and "food is medicine."

I appreciate other authors whose work has contributed to my own. These individuals include Dr. Susanna Czeranko, an amazing researcher who has compiled volumes of naturopathic information into amazing books I was able to use for reference; Jon Rappaport, whose writing and work, which I adore and have been reading for many years, woke me and so many others up to the AIDS lie. His book, *AIDS Inc.*, confirmed my suspicions about viruses.

Thank you, Alec Zeck, for inviting me to present on four panels for "The End of COVID" summit series. It helped me find my voice. You're an inspiration to those searching for answers.

Thank you to the Bigelsen family, including Dr. Harvey (a man I never met, but miss nonetheless). Adam and Josh, by carrying on the love and work of your father, a great man, his memory and influence will last beyond the last star in the sky. Because of you, I look into my microscope in a whole new way. Thank you for your support, kindness, and laughs.

To all the various scientists, journalists, and doctors who constantly question the false narrative of our broken health system, I thank you.

To those who have interviewed me, and continue to pursue the truth with your platforms, thank you.

Mike Stone and Jacob Diaz, thank you for keeping me on my toes. I appreciate your knowledge and wisdom.

Dr. Kirk, thanks for sharing your guidance and wisdom with me when I worked at Pleo Sanum teaching the public about products that most people do not understand.

Reading the wonderful book *Real Food* initially set the stage for me to connect food to health, so I thank Nina Planck, its author, for inspiring my approach to health care.

To the countless naturopaths and true doctors of health that have come before me, I'm honored to stand with you. All your works I hold dear to me and endlessly inspire me to continue to purvey all your messages.

Last, but not least, I am grateful to everyone who strives to be happy and healthy without relying on chemicals and quick fixes. Please continue to have faith in yourself and the choices you make for your family. I applaud and respect you for your effort. You are the hope for humanity's future.

NOTES

FOREWORD

1. 2ndvtrepublic. "COVID-19 and 5G: Connex? (BEINGS OF FREQUENCY)," *Vermont Independent* (March 20, 2020).

INTRODUCTION

Epigraph. B. Stanford Claunch, "How Disease Is Built," an address delivered before the Common Sense Health Club, San Francisco (1923).

ONE: THE DISCOVERY OF "GERMS"

Epigraph. Hugh Desaix Riordan. *Medieval Mavericks, volume 1* (Wichita, KS.: Bio-Communications Press, 1988): p. 5.

1 George E. Billman. " Homeostasis: The Underappreciated and Far Too Often Ignored Central Organizing Principle of Physiology," *Frontiers in Physiology*, vol. 11 (March 10, 2020): p. 200.

2 Theodore H. Tulchinsky. "John Snow, Cholera, the Broad Street Pump: Waterborne Diseases Then and Now," published online, *Case Studies in Public Health* (March 30, 2018): pp. 77–99.

3 H. W. Conn. *The Story of Germ Life* (1898): p. 4.

4 "Friedrich Gustav Jacob Henle," Britannica.com (accessed July 24, 2022).

[5] Patrick Pringle. "The Romance of Modern Science," *Scientific American*, vol. 3, no. 22 (November 1860): p. 346.

[6] *Encyclopaedia Britannica*, first edition (1771).

[7] Émile Duclaux. *Pasteur: The History of a Mind* (1920).

[8] CFH Admin. "Why Does Fermentation Work and How Does It Occur?" culturesforhealth.com (February 3, 2023).

[9] Montague Richard Leverson. "Pasteur the Plagiarist: The Debt of Science to Béchamp," a lecture delivered at Claridge's Hotel in London, England, on May 25, 1911.

[10] From Sir William Osler's lectures on the "Evolution of Modern Medicine," delivered at Yale University in New Haven, CT., in April 1913, for the Silliman Foundation.

[11] Louise Robbins. *Louis Pasteur and the Hidden World of Microbes* (New York: Oxford University Press, 2001): p. 11. Also *see*, Gerald L. Geison. *Private Science of Louis Pasteur* (Princeton, N.J.: Princeton University Press, 1995): p. 179.

[12] Geison: p. 185.

[13] Ibid.: p. 189.

[14] Ibid.: pp. 446–7, 450.

[15] Ibid.: p. 149.

[16] *Pleomorphism* is the occurrence of more than one distinct form of a natural object, such as a crystalline sub-stance, a (supposed) virus, cells in a tumor, or an organism at different stages in its life cycle.

[17] Steven M. Opal. "A Brief History of Microbiology and Immunology," in *Vaccines: A Biography* (New York: Springer, 2010): p. 47.

TWO: THE MAIN CONTENTION OF GERM THEORY

Epigraph. Bartlett Joshua Palmer (1882–1961) is known as the "developer" of chiropractic. His father was the founder.

1 Paul W. Ewald. *Plague Time: The New Germ Theory of Disease* (New York: Anchor Books, 2002): p. 82.

2 Stanford Kingsley Claunch, "How Disease Is Built," an address delivered before the Common Sense Health Club, San Francisco (1923).

3 Inn-Hee Hur. *Korean Medicine: A Holistic Way to Health and Healing* (Seoul, Korea: Seoul Selection, 2013), p. 20–1.

THREE: THE NEGLECTED TERRAIN MODEL OF HEALTH AND HEALING

Epigraph. Harvey Bigelsen. *Holographic Blood: A New Dimension in Medicine* (Nevada City, CA.: Hemobiographic Publications, 2006): p. 29.

1 "About the Foundation,"WestonAPrice.org (accessed November 4, 2024).

2 Mark Jackson, in *The History of Medicine: A Beginner's Guide* (London, U.K.: Oneworld Publications, 2014): p. 151.

3 "Claude Bernard: French Scientist," Britannica.com (accessed April 30, 2024).

4 Claude Bernard. *An Introduction to the Study of Experimental Medicine* (New York: Dover Publications, 2018): p. 88. Originally published in French in 1865.

5 Ibid.: p. 38.

6 Rudolf Virchow. *Inflammation: Irritation and Irritability*, translated M. Félix Pétard (1859).

[7] Fielding H. Garrison. *An Introduction to the History of Medicine: With Medical Chronology, Suggestions for Study, and Bibliographic Data* (Philadelphia, PA.: W.B. Saunders Co., 2001): p. 313.

[8] Alexander Moore. "Hygiene," *Good Health: A Journal of Physical and Mental Culture*, vol. 3 (1871): p. 341.

[9] Ibid.

[10] Rachel Hajar, "The Air of History (Part IV): Great Muslim Physicians Al Rhazes," *Heart Views*, vol. 14, no. 2 (April–June 2013): p. 93.

[11] *Encyclopedia Britannica*, vol 3 (1771): p. 155.

[12] Max von Pettenkofer and Thomas Whiteside Hime. *Cholera: How to Prevent and Resist It* (London, U.K.: Baillière Tindall & Cox, 1883): p. 20.

[13] Ibid.: p. 22.

[14] Ibid.: p. 23.

[15] Seale Harris. "Tuberculosis in the Negro," *Journal of the American Medical Association*, vol. 41, no. 14 (March 1903): p. 60.

[16] Bowery Boys. "The Corona Ash Dump: Brooklyn's Burden on Queens, a Vivid Literary Inspiration and Bleak, Rat-Filled Landscape," boweryboyshistory.com (May 9, 2013).

[17] T. Mitchell Prudden, in *Drinking-Water and Ice Supplies: And Their Relations to Health and Disease* (New York: G.P. Putnam's Sons, 1891): p. 129.

[18] Ibid.: p. 131.

[19] Benedict Lust. *The Naturopath and Herald of Health*, vol. 24 (1919): p. 166.

[20] B. Stanford Claunch, "How Disease Is Built," an address delivered before the Common Sense Health Club, San Francisco (1923).

[21] Sussanna Czeranko, editor. *Origins of Naturopathic Medicine: In Their Own Words* (Portland, OR: NCNM Press, 2013), p. 33.

FOUR: HOW FAITH IN NATURE WAS SUPPLANTED BY FEAR OF NATURE

Epigraph. Albert Schweitzer. *Civilization and Ethics* (1929).

[1] J.M. Peebles. *Vaccination, a Curse and a Menace to Personal Liberty: With Statistics Showing Its Dangers and Criminality* (Battle Creek, MI.: Temple of Health Publishing, 1900): pp. 30–1.

[2] Ibid.

[3] Harold J. Detweiler. "Naturopathy vs. Medicine," *The Naturopath and Herald of Health* (Pune, India: OWPH, 1937).

[4] Hans Knoch, "The Kuhne Cure in *The Naturopath and Herald of Health*, vol.7, no. 2, (Pune: OWPH, 1906) pp. 53–8.

[5] Hereward Carrington. "The Plague in *The Naturopath and Herald of Health*, vol. 14, no 6, (Pune: OWPH, 1909), pp. 353–8.

[6] Ronald Campbell Macfie, in *The Romance of Medicine* (Ithica, NY: Cornell University Library, 1907), p. 136.

[7] Herbert Shelton. *Human Life: It's Philosophy and Laws* (Oklahoma City, OK.: How to Live Publishing, 1928): pp. 189–90.

[8] George Starr White. *Youth Obtained and Retained* (1921).

[9] S.S. Kashaf, D.M. Proctor, C. Deming, et al. "Integrating Cultivation and Metagenomics for a Multi-Kingdom View of Skin microbiome Diversity and Functions. *Natural Microbiology*, vol. 7, 169–79 (December 24, 2022).

[10] Bernhard Päetzold, as cited by Bianca Nogrady. "Biotech Tries Manipulating the Skin Microbiome," *Scientist* (April 18, 2022).

[11] Ed Yong. *I Contain Multitudes: The Microbes Within Us and a Grander View of Life* (New York: Ecco Press, 2018): p. 215.

[12] Fereshteh Mohamadhasani and Mehdi Rahimi. "Grpowth Response and Mycoremediation of Heavy Metals by Fungus *Pleurotus sp.*," *Scientific Reports* (November 19, 2022): article 19947.

[13] Louis Pasteur and Joseph Lister. *Germ Theory and Its Applications to Medicine and on the Antiseptic Principle of the Practice of Surgery* (Amherst, N.Y.: Prometheus Books, 1996): p. 111. Originally published in 1879.

[14] Ibid.: p. 121.

[15] Robert .S. Munford. "Endotoxemia: Menace, Marker, or Mistake? *Journal of Leukocyte Biology*, vol. 100, no. 4 (October 2016): pp. 687–98.

[16] Thomas E. Levy. *Curing the Incurable: Vitamin C, Infectious Diseases, and Toxins, Fourth Edition* (Henderson, NV.: MedFox Publishing, 2002), p. 113.

[17] Rudolf Steiner. "Primary and Secondary Causes and Allopathic Medicine" (1920), in *Viral Illness and Epidemics in the Works of Rudolph Steiner*, edited and translated by

Daniel Hines (Longmont, CO.: Aelzina Books, 2020): p. 104.

18 "Sun Forces and Pathogens" (1921), Ibid.: p. 105.

19 "Pathogens and Illness" (1922), Ibid.: p. 106.

FIVE: THE KEY TO OPTIMAL HEALTH IS WITHIN OUR BODIES

Epigraph. Jesse Mercer Gehman. "The Synthetic Immunization Craze," *Naturopath and Herald of Health*, vol. 41, no. 1 (1937).

1. Antoine Béchamp. *Blood and Its Third Element* (U.S.: Metropolis Ink, 2002): p. 13.
2. Lida H. Mattman. *Cell Wall Deficient Forms: Stealth Pathogens* (Boca Raton, FL.: 2001): p. 2.
3. Béchamp: p. 209.
4. H.W. Wade and C. Manalang. "Fungous Developmental Growth Forms of Bacillus Influenzae: A Preliminary Note," *Journal of Experimental Medicine*, vol. 31, no. 1 (January 1, 1920): pp. 95–103.
5. Milton Wainwright. "Extreme Pleomorphism and the Bacterial Life Cycle: A Forgotten Controversy," *Perspectives in Biology and Medicine*, vol. 40, no. 3 (spring 1997): pp. 407–14.
6. Cornelia Schwerdtle and Franz Arnoul. *Introduction into Darkfield Diagnostics: The Examination of Native Blood According to Prof. Dr. Günther Enderlein* (Germany: Semmelweis-Verlag, 1993): p. 9.

7. Günter Weigel. *A Comprehensive Guide to Sanum Therapy: According to Professor Enderlein* (Hoya, Germany: Semmelweis-Verlag, 2001): pp. 8–17.

8. Lynn Margulis. *Symbiotic Planet: A New Look at Evolution* (New York: Basic Books, 1998).

9. Jeffrey Fisher. "Gaston Naessens and His Cure for Cancer," UnatiranWisdom.com (accessed April 26, 2023).

10. Christopher Bird. *The Persecution and Trial of Gaston Naessens* (Tiburon, CA.: HJ Kramer, 1991): p. 10.

11. Ibid.: p. 11

12. Gerry Vassilatos. "Raymond Rife and His Amazing Microscope," UnariunWisdom.com (accessed January 17, 2025).

13 Royal Rife as cited by R.E. Seidel and M. Elizabeth Winter. "The New Microscopes," *Annual Report of the Board of Regents of the Smithsonian Institution*, vol. 237, no.2 (February 1944).

14. Wilhelm Reich. *The Cancer Biopathy: The Discovery of Orgone, Volume 2* (New York: Orgone Institute Press, 1973): p. 81.

15. Byung-Cheon Lee, et al. "A Hypothesis for a Hidden Circulation System with Cell-Free DNA Molecules, Microvesicles and Microparticles: The Primo Vascular System (Bonghan System), a Putative Acupuncture Meridian System," *Journal of Extracellular Vesicles*. In press (2024).

16. Kyung A. Kang, Claudio Maldonado, and Vitaly Vodyanoy. "Technical Challenges in Current Primo Vascular System Research and Potential Solutions," *Journal of Acupuncture*

and Meridian Studies, vol. 9, no. 6 (December 2016): p. 297e306

17. B. H. Kim. "Sanals and Hematopoiesis," *Journal of Jo Sun Medicine* (1965): pp. 1–6.

18. Royal Lee and William A. Hanson. *Protomorphology: The Principles of Cell Auto-Regulation* (Brookfield, WI.: Lee Foundation for Nutritional Research, 1947). Also see, Royal Lee. *Lectures of Dr. Royal Lee, Volume 1* (Fort Collins, CO.: Selene River Press, 1998): p. 208.

19. August Weisman and Edward Poulton. *Essays upon Heredity and Kindred Biological Problems* (Oxford, U.K.: Clarendon Press, 1891): p. 141.

20. Thorburn Brailsford Robertson. "Experimental Studies on Cellular Multiplication," *Biochemical Journal, vol. 15, no. 5 (1921)*: pp. 612–19.

21. Peter Schneider. "Prof. Enderlein's Research in Today's View: Can His Research Results Be Confirmed with Modern Techniques?" *SANUM-Post* (2001).

22. Cash Asher. *Bacteria Inc.*(Milwaukee, WI.: Lee Foundation for Nutritional Research, 1955): p. 5.

23. William Miller. "Germs . . . Cause of Disease?" *Health Culture* (June 1955): p. 2.

24. A.P. Wood and D.P. Kelly. "Re-classification of Thiobacillus thyasiris as Thibacillus thyasirae comb., nov., an organism exhibiting pleomorphism in response to environmental conditions," *Arch. Microbial.* vol. 159 (1993): pp. 45–7. Also *see*, P.E. Pease and J.E. Tallack. "A permanent endoparasite of man. 1. The silent zoogleal/

symplasm/L-form phas,". *Microbios.* vol. 64 (1990): pp. 173–80.

25. Stuart Grace. "An Open Letter on Pleomorphic Microbiology: Unbundling the Enderlein Legacy," Natural Philosophy Research Group (2001).

26. Lida H. Mattman. *Cell Wall Deficient Forms: Stealth Pathogens* (Boca Raton, FL.: CRC Press, 2000): p. 1.

27. Maria Bleker. *Unappreciated Friend or Unsuspected Foe* (Hoya, Germany: Semmelweis-Verlag, 2004).

SIX: THE IMPORTANCE OF THE EARTH TO OUR TERRAIN

Epigraph. Thich Nhat Hahn. *The World We Have: A Buddhist Approach to Peace and Ecology* (Berkeley, CA.: Parallax Press, 2004): pp. 69–70.

1. Ernst Almquist. "Variation and Life Cycles of Pathogenic Bacteria," *Journal of Infectious Diseases*, vol. 31, no. 5 (November 1922): pp. 483–493.
2. Mark Boyer. "Five Reasons Parasites Are Beneficial to Earth," Science.HowStuffWorks.com (April 16, 2024).
3. Royal Lee. "Primary Cause of Disease," in *Lectures of Dr. Royal Lee, Volume I* (Fort Collins, CO.: Selene River Press, 1998): pp. 34–40.
4. Salma Teimoori, et al. "Heavy Metal Bioabsorption Capacity of Intestinal Helminths in Urban Rats," *Iranian Journal of Public Health*, vol. 43, no. 3 (March 2014): pp. 310–5.

5. Dawn Lester and David Parker. *What Really Makes You Ill?: Why Everything You Thought You Knew about Disease Is Wrong* (United Kingdom: 2019).
6. E.C Rosenow. "Transmutations Within the Streptococcus-Pneumococcus Group," *Journal of Infectious Diseases*, vol. 14, no. 1 (1914): pp.1–32.
7. Richard L. Doty. "Human Pheromones: Do They Exist?" from *Neurobiology of Chemical Communication*, edited by Carla Mucignat-Caretta (Boca Raton, FL.: CRC Press/Taylor & Francis, 2014). See also, Richard L. Doty. *The Great Pheromone Myth* (Baltimore, MD.: Johns Hopkins University Press, 2010).
8. Martin Blank and Reba Goodman, "DNA Is a Fractal Antenna in Electromagnetic Fields," *International Journal of Radiation Biology*, vol. 87, no. 4 (2011): pp. 409–15. Also see: Grazyna Fosar and Franz Bludorf. "Scientists Prove DNA Can Be Reprogrammed by Words and Frequencies," sikhnet.com (September 12, 2011).
9. Richard Bright. "The Rhythmic Sound of Living Cells," interaliamag.org (September 2015).
10. Michel Gauquelin. *The Scientific Basis of Astrology*, translated by James Hughes (New York: Stein and Day, 1969): p. 203.
11. Michel Gauquelin. *The Cosmic Clocks: From Astrology to a Modern Science* (Washington, D.C.: Henry Regnery Co., 1967): p. 211.
12. Ibid.: p. 186.
13. Ibid.,: p. 223.

14. James Clark. *The Sanative Influence of Climate, third edition* (Philadelphia, PA: A. Waldie, 1841).

SEVEN: HOW DO VIRUSES FIT IN THE TERRAIN MODEL

Epigraph. Johann Wolfgang von Goethe. *Aphorisms on the Theory of Nature and Science* (1869).

1. Torsten Engelbrecht and Claus Köhnlein. *Virus Mania: How the Medical Industry Continually Invents Epidemics, Making Billion-Dollar Profits at Our Expense* (Bloomington, IN.: Trafford Publishing, 2007).
2. Janet M. Arce (graduate thesis). "The Effect of Natural and Synthetic Prostaglandins on Erythropoiesis in the Mouse," New York University (September 1982).
3. Tobias I. Baskin, et al. "Sample Preparation for Scanning Electron Microscopy: The Surprising Case of Freeze Drying from Tertiary Butanol," *Microscopy Today*, vol. 22, no. 3 (2014): pp. 36–9.
4. Peter H. Duesberg, *Inventing the AIDS Virus* (Washington, D.C.: Regnery Pub., 1997).
5. Michiel Pegtel and Stephen J. Gould. "Exosomes," *Annual Review of Biochemistry*, vol. 88 (June 2019): pp. 487–514.
6. Stefan Lanka. "The Misconception Called Virus," *Wissenschafftplus* (January 2020): pp. 2–12.
7. Dawn Lester and David Parker. *What Really Makes You Ill? Why Everything You Thought You Knew about Disease Is Wrong* (United States: Dawn Lester & David Parker, 2019).
8. Thomas S. Cowan and Sally Fallon Morell, in *The Contagion Myth: Why Viruses (Including "Coronavirus") Are*

Not the Cause of Disease (New York, NY: Skyhorse Publishing, 2020): p. 71.

9. Harvey Bigelsen. Lecture to the 2006 conference of the International Association of Biological Dental Medicine.
10. "History—Günther Enderlein," BRMI.online (accessed April 7, 2025).
11. It is impossible to use a darkfield microscope (or fluoroscope) for this purpose because this instrument, which is designed for observing the internal structure of an opaque object (such as the living body), functions by means of X-rays.

EIGHT: FLAWS IN MODERN MEDICAL SCIENCE AND ITS INDUSTRIALIZATION

Epigraph. Theodore Fox was the editor-in-chief of *The Lancet* from 1944–1964. From his 1965 Harveian Oration, "Purposes of Medicine," Royal College of Physicians of London.

1. G. M. Edelman, et al. "Structural Differences among Antibodies of Different Specificities," *Proceedings of the National Academy of Sciences*, vol. 47, no. 11 (November 15, 1961): pp. 1751–8.
2. W. H. Manwaring. "The Basic Concepts of Immunity," *Journal of Immunology*, vol. 12, no. 3 (April 1, 1926), pp. 177–84.
3. Mary Holland, et al. "Unanswered Questions from the Vaccine Injury Compensation Program: A Review of Compensated Cases of Vaccine-Induced Brain Injury,"

May 10, 2011, *Pace Environmental Law Review*, vol. 28, no. 2 (May 10, 2011), pp. 480–531.

4. Torsten Engelbrecht and Köhnlein Claus. *Virus Mania: How the Medical Industry Continually Invents Epidemics, Making Billion-Dollar Profits at Our Expense* (Bloomington, IN.: Trafford Publishing, 2007).

5. R. E. Brandman. "The Medical Trust Busy Again," *Naturopath and Herald of Health*, vol. 18, no. 11 (1913), p. 724.

6. Bernard Lust. Editorial, *Naturopath and Herald of Health* (1907).

7. José Martí. *José Martí: Selected Writings*, edited and translated by Esther Allen (New York: Penguin Books, 2002), p. 133.

8. David Weir and Mark Schapiro. *Circle of Poison: Pesticides and People in a Hungry World* (San Francisco, CA.: Institute for Food and Development Policy, 1981), p. 8.

9. Randall Fitzgerald. *The Hundred-Year Lie: How to Protect Yourself from the Chemicals That Are Destroying Your Health* (New York: Plume, 2007), p. 20.

10. Richard Gerber. *Vibrational Medicine: The #1 Handbook of Subtle-Energy Therapies* (Rochester, VT: Bear & Company, 2001).

NINE: KEEPING THE BALANCE OF THE TERRAIN

Epigraph. Louise Lust. "The Curative Agency of Water and Herbs for Treatment of Fever," *Naturopath*, vol. 28 (1923): p. 437.

1. Reimar Banis. *New Life Through Energy Healing: The Atlas of Psychosomatic Energetics* (Nevada City, CA.: Artemis Books, 2008). pp. 62–4.
2. Ibid.
3. Ibid.
4. Claude Bernard. *An Introduction to the Study of Experimental Medicine* (Garden City, N.Y.: Dover Publications, 1957), translation by Henry Copley Greene. Originally published in French in 1865 and English in 1927.
5. Rudolf Steiner and Christian von Arnim, *Nutrition: Food, Health and Spiritual Development* (London, U.K.: Rudolf Steiner Press, 2009), p. 172.
6. Sharyn Wynters and Burton Goldburg. *The Pure Cure: A Complete Guide to Freeing Your Life from Dangerous Toxins* (Berkeley, CA.: Soft Skull Press, 2012).
7. C.S. Carr. "Vaccination Wholly Empirical," *Naturopath and Herald of Health*, vol. 8, no. 7 (1907) : p. 220.

TEN: TERRAIN-MODEL THERAPEUTICS

Epigraph. Harvey Bigelsen. *Doctors Are More Harmful Than Germs: How Surgery Can Be Hazardous to Your Health—And What to Do About It, Illustrated Edition* (Berkeley, CA.: North Atlantic Books, 2011): p. 29.

ELEVEN: OVERCOMING MALNUTRITION CAUSED BY DEFICITS IN OUR FARMING PRACTICES

Epigraph. Benedict Lust. Editorial, *Herald of Health* (February 1921).

1. Royal Lee. *Lectures of Dr. Royal Lee, Volume I*, compiled and edited by Mark R. Anderson (Selene River Press, Inc, 1998): p. 39.
2. Ibid.: p. 3.
3. Frederick Robert Klenner, "The Treatment of Poliomyelitis and Other Virus Diseases with Vitamin C," *South Med Surg.* 111, no. 7 (July 1949): pp. 209–214.
4. Thomas E. Levy. *Curing the Incurable: Vitamin C, Infectious Diseases, and Toxins* (Philadelphia, PA: Xlibris, 2002).
5. T.W.B. Osborn and J.H.S. Gear. "Possible Relation Between Ability to Synthesize Vitamin C and Reaction to Tubercle Bacillus: Semantic Scholar," Nature, vol.145, no. 3686 (June 22, 1940): p. 974.
6. Paula Baillie-Hamilton. *Toxic Overload: A Doctor's Plan for Combating the Illnesses Caused by Chemicals in Our Foods, Our Homes, and Our Medicine Cabinets* (New York: Penguin, 2005).
7. Luoping Zhang, et al. "Exposure to Glyphosate-based Herbicides and Risk for Non-Hodgkin Lymphoma: A Meta-analysis and Supporting Evidence," *Mutation Research*, vol. 781 (July–September, 2019): pp. 186–206.
8. AGDaily staff. "The List of Organic Pesticides Approved by the USDA," AGDaily.com (January 15, 2025).
9. Raymond Francis. *The Great American Health Hoax: The Surprising Truth About How Modern Medicine Keeps You Sick—How to Choose a Healthier, Happier, and Disease-Free Life* (Deerfield Beach, FL.: Health Communications, Inc., 2014): p. 148.

TWELVE: DETOXIFICATION AND REDUCING THE BODY'S WORKLOAD

Epigraph. Sherry A. Rogers. *Tired or Toxic? A Blueprint for Health* (Syracuse, N.Y.: Prestige Publishing, 1990): p. 85.

THIRTEEN: YOU ARE THE SUM OF YOUR ANCESTORS' MICROBIOMES AND TERRAIN

Epigraph. Henry Lindlahr. *Nature Cure: Philosophy and Practice Based on the Unity of Disease and Cure* (Chicago, IL.: Nature Cure Publishing Company, 1922): p. 529.

1. "You've Been Lied to about Genetics," YouTube video, posted by SubAnima, January 20, 2023.
2. Weston A. Price. *Nutrition and Physical Degeneration* (La Mesa, CA.: Price-Pottenger Nutrition Foundation, 2020).
3. Abraham Wasserstein. *Galen's Commentary on the Hippocratic Treatise, Airs, Waters, Places: In the Hebrew Translation of Solomon ha-Me'ati* (Jerusalem, Israel: Israel Academy of Sciences and Humanities, 1982).
4. Vincenzo Monda, et al. "Exercise Modifies the Gut Microbiota with Positive Health Effects," *Oxidative Medicine and Cellular Longevity* 2017 (March 5, 2017): 28357027. Also *see*, Ask the Doctors. "Time Spent Outdoors Helpful to Gut Microbiome," UCLAHealth.org (January 21, 2025).
5. William Trebing. *Goodbye Germ Theory: Ending a Century of Medical Fraud* (Bloomington, IN.: Xlibris Corporation, 2006): p. 170.

FOURTEEN: BREAK THE SPELL OF GERM THEORY EVERYWHERE

Epigraph. Simon Louis Katzoff. *Timely Truths on Human Health* (1921).

1. Transcript of keynote address to 2015 Appalachian Energy Summit. "Robert F. Kennedy, Jr., on Choosing to Preserve Our Assets," *Appalachian Today* (August 14, 2015).
2. William Freeman Havard. *The Treatment of Acute Diseases* (1921).
3. Louis Kuhne. *The New Science of Healing: Or the Doctrine of the Unity of Diseases Forming the Basis of a Uniform Method of Cure Without Medicines or Operations* (1899).
4. Prem Anjali. "Enlightenment: An Unlearning Process—A Conversation with Marianne Williamson," *Integral Yoga Magazine* (winter 2013).
5. John Ryder. "How Hypnosis Can Heal the Body," *Psychology Today*, blog (October 19, 2010).

AFTERWORD

1. Benedict Lust. *Herald of Health* (1921): p. 21.
2. Melvin E. Page and H. Leon Abrams, Jr. *Your Body Is Your Best Doctor* (Bloomington, IN.: iUniverse, 1972): p. 3. Originally published in 1960 as *Health versus Disease.*
3. Ibid.: p. 38.
4. Louise Lust. "How to Avoid Pain and Sickness," *Naturopath Magazine*, vol. 16 (1911): p. 99.
5. James C. Thomson. *The Heart: The Prevention and Cure of Cardiac Conditions* (London, U.K.: Thorsons, 1939): p. 65.

RESOURCES

Marizelle Arce, N.D.
https://terraindoctor.com
Email: dr.mari@terraindoctor.com

Please come to my website, to learn more about what you can personally do for your health and the environment.

ABOUT THE AUTHOR

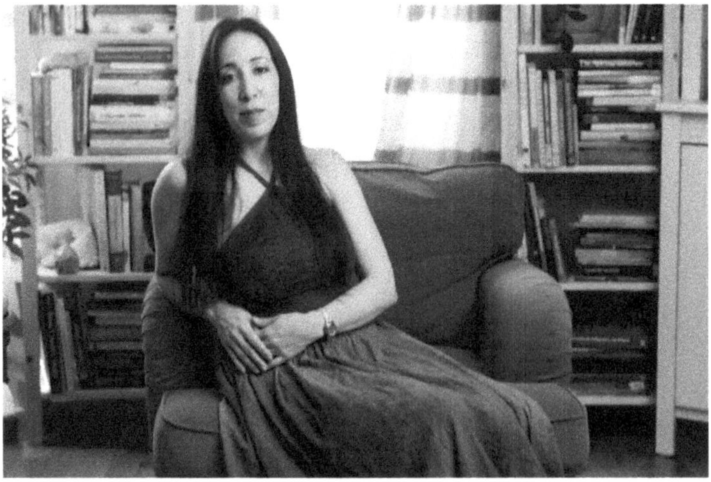

Marizelle Arce, N.D., is a pioneering naturopathic terrain doctor, certified kinesiologist, and nutrition expert. Since 2015, She has been the leader of the Westchester chapter of the Weston A. Price Foundation. She also runs a private healthcare practice in New York State.

Dr. Arce holds a bachelor's degree from Stony Brook University and a doctor of naturopathic medicine degree from the University of Bridgeport, College of Naturopathic Medicine. At U.B., she specialized in nutrition and food education for degenerative diseases as well as preventative health, and became interested in ancestral healthcare.

Over the past sixteen years, Dr. Arce has helped countless individuals from all walks of life overcome unexplainable health issues. Her tireless determination to seek answers to their unsolved questions has driven her to find solutions for even the most puzzling cases. She has also overcome health issues of her own that were initially considered idiopathic (or, arising from an unidentifiable origin) through the application of findings from her avid research.

As a medical student, Dr. Arce worked for Pleomorphic Sanum, a company whose guiding philosophy filled in some of the blanks regarding questions that none of her schooling had answered for her, in particular, the true cause of diseases. The greatest answer of all was the symbiotic relationship of humans with what the world popularly refers to as *germs*. Unlike most of her classmates, Dr. Arce wholeheartedly embraced classical naturopathy and her new understanding of microorganisms.

After completing her medical degree, Dr. Arce continued pursuing her passion for traditional therapies and modes of treatment. She studied and became certified in herbology, iridology, applied kinesiology, live blood cell analysis, and physiotherapy. Armed with this knowledge, she opened her private practice in 2007, intent on bringing her innovative approach to every person seeking care from her.

Dr. Arce is a proponent of sustainable farming done without pesticides or synthetic fertilizers, clean water, and an unpolluted environment, the use of nontoxic building materials, and strict adherence to traditional dietary principles; as well as of the avoidance of vaccines and pharmaceutical agents. Her health-care practice is drugless.

Dr. Arce resides in Westchester County, New York. She is married with two children.

www.ingramcontent.com/pod-product-compliance
Lightning Source LLC
Chambersburg PA
CBHW052027030426
42337CB00027B/4898
9798992628500